SHRED

Removing the layers to find your true purpose

By Sandra D. Cleveland, PhD, MSN, RN, NETA-CGEI

Copyright Notice © 2019 Sandra D. Cleveland.

All rights reserved, including any right to reproduce this book or portion thereof in any form whatsoever.

This book is designed to provide accurate and authoritative information with regard to the subject matter covered. It is sold with the understanding that there is not a professional consulting engagement. If legal or other expert advice or assistance in required please consult with a licensed professional in your area.

For information on bulk orders to have Sandra D. Cleveland speak at your event please contact Sandra D. Cleveland at tribeconsulting4u@gmail.com

Table of Contents

Shred: Removing The Layers To Find Your True Purpose
By Sandra D. Cleveland, Phd, Msn, Rn, Neta-Cgei 3

From Broken To Purpose: How Caring For Others Helped Me Overcome Abuse And Trauma
By Dawn Bork 19

Feathers May Fall, But Wings Will Fly
By Charlene Harrod-Owuamana, Aas Lpn Hbot Wc 33

Chozen: Discovering Purpose In Life And In Nursing
By Onissa S. Mitchell, Msn, Rn, Aprn, Fnp-C 45

Dark Beginnings Don't Have To Mean Dark Endings: Women On Purpose
By Lola Olarunfemi 62

The Blooming Gift
By Malina Spears, Lpn 74

Sowing The Seeds Of Purpose
By Kecia Hayslett, Rn, Htc 85

Push Past Your Fear And Find Your Purpose: A Woman's Anthology To Power
By Tina Marie Payne, Msn, Rn 97

Beginnings: An Antology for Woman Acknowledging Their Gifts
By Willa Smiley, Msn, Med, RN, Ccm, Lnc 113

Against The Odds
By Kerine Dent-Alston, Rn 126

SHRED

Removing the layers to find your true purpose

Acknowledgement

To the Wonderful Counselor, for showing me I would not be blessed until I became a blessing…

My husband, for helping me balance reality and my dreams…

My awesome kids – my faith spoken through their voices…

My parents – my original earthly faith-builders…

For those who questioned my abilities – you helped me find my perseverance, my truth and show that *if I'm aligned with HIM in my purpose, I can not be stopped.*

SHRED

Removing the layers to find your true purpose

By Sandra D. Cleveland, PhD, MSN, RN, NETA-CGEI

I have a couple of secrets I want to share with you. My first secret is although I always steered towards helping people, I was a sports nut and wanted to help people through something like sports medicine – nursing was not even on the radar for me at the time. I've also had a secret ambition to write a novel. I would have chapters themed around song titles of my favorite music group (Earth, Wind & Fire) or write about stories related to my love of sports and the lessons we can learn from them. I wanted to create characters that were larger than life, dealing with life scenarios where the reader would sit and say, "what a great experience," or "I can't believe that happened!" I used to think that I have read books all my life to escape; rather, I have actually used books to run to experiences that I thought I could never have. As I sit here sharing my story, I find that the analogy that really relates to my life is exercise – or more specifically, an activity called shredding.

Physical inactivity and a sedentary lifestyle are contributing factors to the scope and breadth of chronic diseases and illness experienced worldwide. Studies have shown that physical activity, across all lifespans, is positively associated with a reduction in cardiovascular disease, stroke, hypertension, type 2 diabetes and obesity, as well as an improvement in anxiety and depression (Nelson et al., 2007). When I think about how this relates to my journey towards my purpose, I can see that the periods in my life where I felt unfocused or misguided amounted to a sedentary attempt to purpose. I had to understand and stay motivated to implement a purpose driven exercise plan.

What is a SHRED? Shredding is a type of exercise regimen that is focused on the goals of weight loss, body fat percentage loss and muscle strength and definition. Shredding integrates the components of fitness: strength, flexibility, balance and power. Those who work out in the gym or with a personal trainer are bound to have heard the term "shred" used at one point or another. The definition itself focuses on the goals; but one also must realize that there are adjustments (major or minor) that need to be made for success to be achieved. It's always easier to state, "I want to lose weight" rather than "I want to lose 20 lbs. in the next 8 weeks." However, by generalizing the goal, you don't provide enough direction or strategy to be successful. An initial portion of this purpose-driven exercise plan – what I'll refer to as my shred – came from a place of reflection. Reflective practice is an important concept to incorporate. During a shred, athletes must pay attention to the core of their body, identify things they must give up in order to move forward. Like a shred, I share experiences that created my core beliefs, showed instances where I plateaued and times where I needed to release items in order to move forward.

CORE. Growing up in suburban America, I was typically living the life of what Shonda Rhimes identifies in the acknowledgement in her book, *The Year of Yes* as F.O.D. (first, only, different). However, I wanted to believe otherwise. I admittedly thought I was part of the group – thought that even though I was African American in a primarily Caucasian environment, I was truly accepted for what I brought to the table and for who I was. I mean, I was a good student and athlete and followed the rules. My parents are great people…they guided me, took us to church, worked hard and did well in their respective fields.

A couple of incidents in school and at home reminded me that I was truly F.O.D. When we moved from an urban area to Cincinnati, the first incident of blatant dislike for our family became evident. We lived next door to a family where the dad was a cop and they owned a German Shepherd. Their yard was fenced (the only one of the neighboring houses with one). Anytime we went near the fence, the dad often yelled at us. We weren't doing anything particularly wrong – we were just kids of 6-8 years old who played with the other kids in the neighborhood. One day, we were playing Frisbee and the Frisbee went into the yard. We did knock on the door, and he wouldn't get the Frisbee for us. So we tried to get it ourselves – the dad decided to let the dog out after us. We were terrified and didn't understand (when everyone else around us got along just fine) why he would do such a thing.

We moved to Michigan when my dad was transferred in his job. It was often just my younger brother Jim and I as the only African Americans in our respective grades going throughout elementary school. The African American population doubled when we got to high school…there was another African American brother and sister who attended as well. So, now we had one African American student per grade.

The first incident happened in 7th grade. I was sitting at a table with a couple of classmates in the school library. While I don't remember the full discussion, it was based on who liked who in the class….you know, the "Lisa likes Mike, but Mike likes Julie" type of discussion. One of the boys stated that someone liked me, but wouldn't tell the name – however, the bit of excitement that I felt was soon smashed when the other classmate indicated, "monkeys at the zoo are liked, too." Not since we lived in Cinci, next to our racist cop neighbor, had someone blatantly showed out like that. At this point, I left the library, visibly upset and hurt that someone would say that to me. I didn't know where to go and just sat on the steps. The class bell rang soon thereafter and unfortunately, although a number of teachers and students passed by, most did not stop to see why I was so upset. Thankfully, a good friend of mine at the time sat with me – he listened to me share the incident and comforted me.

There have been other events in my life that made me question my worth. One was my first marriage. I met him in college during my freshman year and thought he was a good guy – we were at a university that, at the time, had a low percentage of minorities on campus. On top of that, both of us were in fields where we were F.O.D. That appealed to me, because we could share our feelings and relate to each other. However, I experienced some incidents with him that raised red flags for me. The "Catch-22" in my mind was that not only was I F.O.D. for Caucasians, but I learned I was F.O.D. from other African Americans who lived in cities. How do you reconcile that you belong when everyone you encounter is telling you that you don't fit? You hang on to the one who appears to accept you for who you are – plus, I guess I gained some cred, because he came from a city, as well.

We ended up marrying after college – and unfortunately, the red flags that I ignored while dating could not be ignored now. I was often isolated from my friends and family. I often had to be with his family, who extolled him for almost any reason, reminding me how "lucky" I was to be chosen by him. As the marriage progressed, we did the expected things couples were supposed to do – but on the inside, I was becoming utterly miserable and depressed. When you think of abuse, you may think of physical or loud verbal incidents. But this was more insidious – the words used to converse with me often made me question myself and keep me in an unhealthy place: body, mind and spirit. When I look back in hindsight, I allowed him to use his words to pull me away from my purpose. I finally hit rock bottom and just couldn't take it anymore. I requested marriage counseling a number of times, but everything was always my fault. Finally, I gave myself approval to seek counseling for just me.

Counseling was freeing. I could just TALK. For a while, most of my discussions focused on the things I did wrong (perceived and real). But what I realized as I continued my sessions is that he could control me because I relinquished my power to him. Sometimes you just need someone who is not a friend or family member to provide and question your perspective and help you understand that you have validity in the world. Counseling slowly taught me how to regain my voice. To regain my spiritual side, I joined a church (I grew up as an active Christian, but did not practice much during this marriage).

PLATEAU (2nd component of the shred). I call these stories part of the plateau. In a shred, there are times that you are stuck in moving towards your goals. There are incidents from an educational perspective that made me question my purpose. I always did well in school – mostly A's and B's. However, when I was working to complete each stage of my education, there were people who doubted my intent or my abilities to complete the programs. One big incident occurred when I worked on my PhD.

By this time, I remarried (it was a number of years later), gained my "instant gift from earth" (my stepson) and was pregnant.

During this time, I experienced a difficult and painful pregnancy early on, and as a result, placed on bed rest for 7 months for the sake of both the baby and me. The doctor told me to put my affairs in place before I went on bed rest. I went to the university and submitted (and had received written approval) for a medical and academic leave of absence, which would keep me out for the full academic year. After having the baby, I was scheduled to attend the next academic year. However, the dean for the program decided to count the time that I was off against the time allotted to complete the program (even with their approval), and removed me from the program.

I was devastated – I had successfully completed all of the coursework and one of the defenses that would allow me to then work on my dissertation. How the heck does that happen?!? But this time, I did not allow this person to fully take my power. I immediately called another university that evening, transferred any courses I could and started with that program. There were only so many of the courses approved for transferring over to the new university. As a result, I had to take about 12-13 additional courses before I could then work on my dissertation (a totally different topic, but more aligned with what I wanted to do). I would go to Starbuck's at 4:30 am every day to work on that dissertation – playing the singing duo Mary Mary's song "Go Get It" as my theme. On March 7, 2014 – 14 years after I started – I walked across the stage with my family witnessing the announced words "Dr. Sandra Cleveland." I was proud because I made it in spite of the naysayers, critics and detractors.

I have had a number of tests and testimonies, but if you'll allow me, let me concentrate on 2 dates - January 19 and August 3 - that tie into two key events in my life. My world would change unequivocally 16 years ago on Jan 19th at 5:30 am…it is forever etched in my mind and heart. That's the day I got a knock on my door, with a policeman on the other end. My first thought was, "what'd I do?" But I was asleep, so that wasn't it...The officer proceeded to give me the news that my brother was in a car accident and didn't make it. His accident was literally 3 minutes from my house. Jim was my "big/little brother" – he was the life of the party and could sell anything. We drove each other crazy, but we loved each other and always had each other's backs. Having to follow the kind officer to my parents' house to share the news was the most heart-wrenching moment in my life. On top of this, my father was diagnosed with prostate cancer about a month after we lost my brother. I didn't want to question God but did it a lot, hoping my brother was okay in heaven and my dad would beat cancer (he did).

My other test came a few years later. I was 3 months pregnant and constantly in pain. I knew I had fibroids. Fibroids are non-cancerous tumors with an unknown cause. It is a condition common in African American women. The pain became persistent and relentless. Finally, on August 3, my OB-GYN stated I needed to go on bed rest as I was at a higher risk due to my age, and the fibroids were growing along with the baby. The fibroids grew so large (about the size of softballs) that they were competing with the baby for blood flow and causing the severe pain. I was an active person – often worked a couple of jobs, worked out, along with the responsibilities of a wife and stepmom. But for the next 7 months, I was only allowed to sit up at a 30 degree angle in bed and restricted to the bathroom and kitchen for short amounts of time each day. In order not to harm the baby, I could only take Tylenol. I normally have a pretty good tolerance for pain – but having pain this long without real relief took a toll on my husband, son, my parents and me. My husband and parents were troopers – there were days where all I could do was cry. They covered the tasks that needed to be done. My mom often let me use her shoulder to cry on – for this I was really thankful. During this time, I prayed often to help me see that things would be okay.

As the months passed, the baby grew healthy and big. I ended up going into the hospital to have my baby two weeks later than the due date. I was in labor for over 24 hours before being brought to the hospital, but my baby didn't want to leave the current residence. I actively labored for another 14 hours, but because the baby's heart kept slowing down, an emergency caesarian section was performed. Remember earlier when I said I wanted to concentrate on the two dates? Well, my beautiful baby girl was born on January 19 at approximately 5:30 am – *4 years to the hour when I lost my brother.* I realized that God had shown me that everything was going to be just fine.

RESIGNATION to REALIZATION (3RD component of the shred). In the shred, the athlete has to be on a "clean" diet – no foods that include preservatives. This often means that the athlete has to give up a number of food types in order to move forward. I equate this idea with episodes of job resignations…let me explain.

I often peruse social media outlets such as Instagram, SnapChat and Facebook. On this particular morning, a post was placed in a group page, with thousands of members, where the post writer posed the question "how many weeks resignation do you have to give?" When the thread reached me, there were already hundreds of responses to this individual's question, which ranged from "a couple of weeks" to "a month." However, this got me to thinking, how much time do I REALLY spend on my resignations based on the definitions above? According to Henry David Thoreau, "What is called Resignation is really confirmed Desperation"…I found this to be true.

The act of writing the resignation letter, in itself, takes as short as 15 minutes to over a week. But I realized something…my frustration at my previous employment was not so much based on the first definition, but allowing myself to <u>really</u> review my mind and my heart as it related to my role. I've done some soul-searching to note that I lived my resignations easily over 4-6 months. That's a LONG time to take oneself through the process of the realization of the desired role vs. the actualized role in the organization; the frustration of living in the dual roles; and the moment where you want to actively realign purpose with the desired roles by taking a leap. WHEW!

For instance, the last couple of roles I had were, I thought, my "dream jobs." I was probably like you with a new job – excited, nervous and ready to put my best foot forward in being indispensable to the organization. My plan was to be with the organizations until I retired…sharing my skills and gifts, actually being recognized for my contributions and steadily moving up in the organization. But God had other plans for me…

When I reflect on my resignations, I found that I was able to share these gifts – there was initial acceptance of these gifts and there was organizational recognition of the ways these gifts translated into things needed to meet the organization's strategic plan. But what tended to happen, after the first couple of years, was that I was not welcomed to share my gifts any further. For instance, one of my talents as a faculty member was mentoring faculty into their new roles. I loved seeing how I could move people from just surviving the organizational nuances, but really starting to thrive in their gifts, thereby finding their niche. The issue in doing this face-to-face all of the time was that we often had conflicting schedules and could not meet as often as both parties desired. I created an avatar-guided Online Orientation for Nursing and Allied Health Professions Faculty, accommodating diverse schedules and helping adjunct faculty feel more engaged in the orientation process. It included topics such as faculty development, future teaching opportunities and FAQ. The project was publicly recognized at the university and also received a stipend to attend and present at conference proceedings. I found out, through my journey, that the letters I had to write were in fact NOT resignation letters to the organization, but acceptance letters of the skills and abilities that were uniquely me and not being used to the fullest. As the actor Michael J. Fox stated during his battle with Parkinson's Disease, "Acceptance doesn't mean resignation; it means understanding that something is what it is and there's got to be a way through it."

FLEXIBILITY (4th component of shred). Flexibility can be applied a few ways for a shred. An athlete needs to be flexible with exercise times; an athlete also needs to incorporate exercises in his/her routine to develop flexibility. I have made changes in many areas of my world to be able to share my God-given ability to mentor others in completing their goals and dreams. This is the year I promised I would say "yes, Lord" and make the leaps I needed for me to live my authentic life. But then I found a lump today... and nobody knows (except you, my new friends).

As a nurse, you would think very clearly that you should know the next steps…you have the knowledge and know what actions you should take. But when it becomes YOU and you are worried on the potential terminology that will be attached to the small mass, it becomes a different story, doesn't it? So, I find myself in limbo (on a mental commercial break, if you will) while I work through the emotions of uncertainty. The "woulda, shoulda, coulda" statements are making their attempt to infiltrate my mind and my spirit. What I continue to wonder is, "why the year that I finally make the leap?" But then I remember Ephesians 4:29 => *Do not let any unwholesome talk come out of your mouths, but only what is helpful for building others up according to their needs that it may benefit those who listen*. I have worked diligently to weave my mentoring throughout all areas of my life…including the times of uncertainty. When the proverbial "test becomes a testimony" is no longer just a religious cliché becomes an important promise and an opportunity to truly "reach one, teach one."

It is so important in your shred to identify how you gain flexibility; release items in your life to move forward on your goals; understand that plateaus do happen. Use these as well as your past experiences and your values (your core) to help with the uncertainties in your life and conquer the deferred dreams and decisions you have or want to make. I share the following:

- Be vulnerable… you don't have to have it all together. Be willing to share your fears and feelings, and quick to acknowledge your mistakes.
- Once you've acknowledged your mistakes, FORGIVE YOURSELF and OTHERS. You need to create this freedom so that you can focus on the task at hand.

- Never stop growing – allow yourself to stretch outside of your comfort zone.

- Distractions can happen and dreams can be temporarily deferred, but work to live your purpose in whatever the situation.

So today, I continue to vow and take the leaps I promised and deal with the lumps in life. I will continue to use the God-given gifts and talents bestowed on me, even in uncertain circumstances. And yes, I did make my appointment.

Conclusion: Health, education, family and FAITH have been elements interwoven throughout my life tapestry. There have been times when I have embraced or denied these threads, but I now realize that these 4 threads are braided together in my life tapestry – and if any one of these areas aren't addressed or denied, then the consequences are felt by myself or those closest to me. In fact, Philippians 4:13 is a philosophy I currently strive to live by - "I can do all things in Him who strengthens me." I believe these threads align with my purpose – and I challenge you to reflect on and speak to a Higher Power about incidents in your life to help you live your purpose. I realize that different people have been brought to me for a "reason, season, or lifetime"…and I continue to look for the lessons from them to apply to my life. Isn't it funny how the truth became definitely larger than any fictional story that I could ever conjure up?

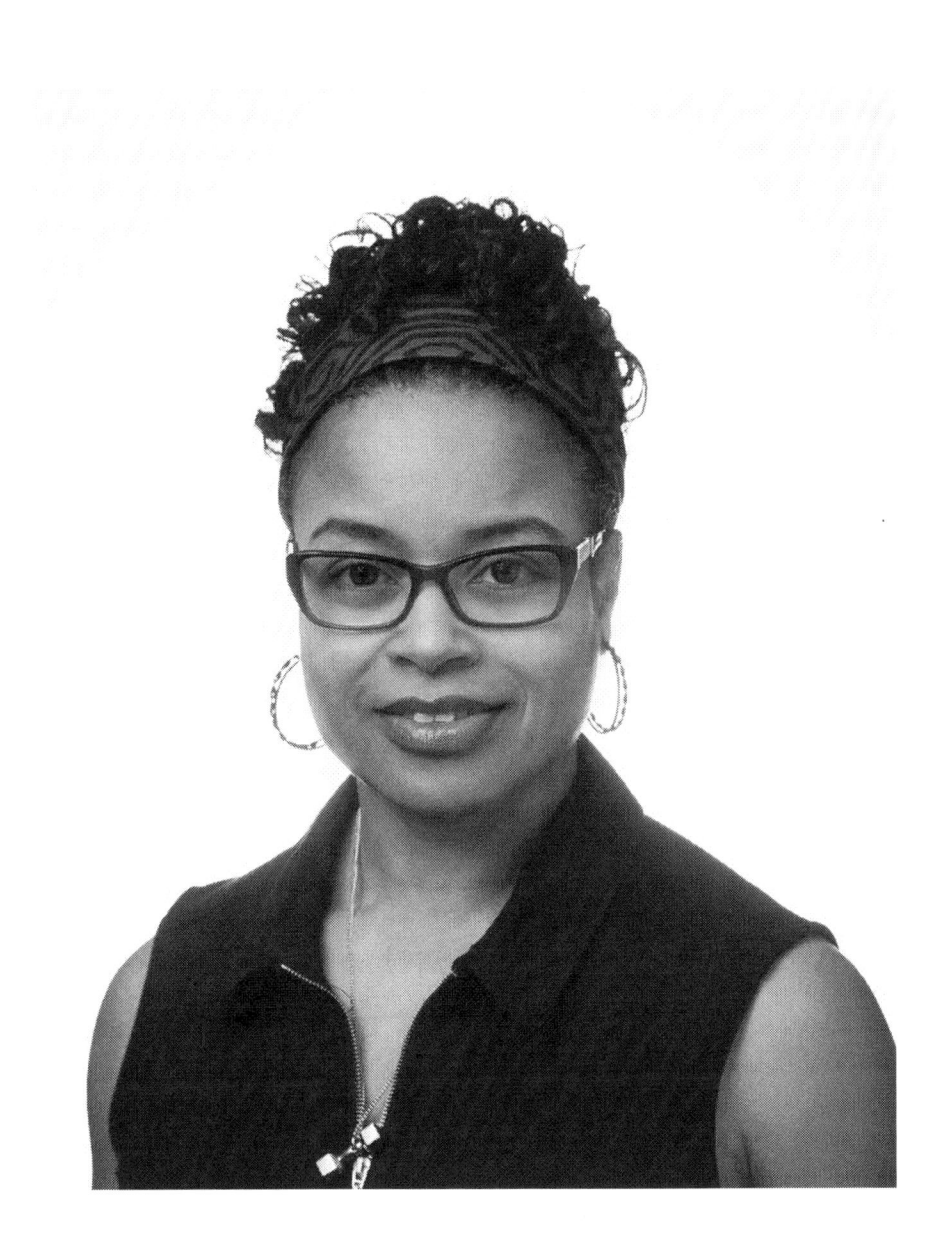

Acknowledgements

I give thanks to God for never leaving nor forsaking me. I thank the many people he placed in my life which kept me grounded and on course to overcome the many obstacles faced along the way.

To my children Karen, Jamal, Raven and Maddie it was your unconditional love that made all the difference and gave me the strength to keep going despite the many times I wanted to give up. You guys are my first loves.

To my husband Joe, thank you for your love and support that you've given so unselfishly. I love you.

FROM BROKEN TO PURPOSE
How caring for others helped me overcome abuse and trauma

By Dawn Bork

Finding purpose in life, and living out that purpose for the good of others, is the ultimate sacrifice. Living life can be challenging and downright unfair at times. There is a saying, "hurt people hurt others." The meaning became very clear to me when I began listening to and watching prison stories. The majority of people serving time in prison came from similar backgrounds as me: Mental, physical, sexual and emotional abuse, including abandonment by a parent. It's a viscous cycle that continues for generations if not dealt with properly. Although I'm thankful I eluded a life of crime due to unresolved hurt, I couldn't help but wonder how and why.

When I was just 2 years old, my two siblings and I were placed in foster care in the state of Wisconsin. My mother and father were having problems regarding my mother's drinking, hanging out in bars, getting arrested and leaving us with neighbors for days at a time. My father, only in his early 20s, couldn't leave his job to take care of and support us. We had no other family living in Wisconsin at the time. My dad called his sister and asked her to fly to Wisconsin and take us back home to South Carolina with her. I remember crying for my parents and wondering why they had to leave us. My dad's family tried to console me, but because I was so young, it was hard to accept anything when all I wanted was my mom and dad. My siblings and I would live the next 5 years without seeing either of our parents on a daily basis.

I remember my aunt and uncle as loving and nurturing to my siblings and I. I always felt safe and loved. I credit this love that my aunt and uncle showed my siblings and me for how my story turned out. My aunt would always say when a person is down, you don't kick him/her further down. She always showed us how to treat others through her own actions. People who knew my aunt loved her. Another of my dad's sisters had us in church at an early age. I didn't always understand what was going on because I was so young. I do feel that having that exposure to God at such a young age has been my saving grace. I don't attend church as I should, but I do believe in God and it is my faith in Him that I know, without a doubt, has brought me this far.

By 8 years old, I was emotionally, mentally, sexually and physically abused. I longed for my mom to take me away and protect me. The more I longed for my mom, the more depressed I became. My mother made no effort to contact my siblings or me. When I was 14 years old I remember telling my dad that I wanted to die, because of the trauma of all the abuse I had suffered (plus the abandonment). If living life the way I was forced to live it was all there was, I'd rather be dead. I couldn't understand why my mother abandoned me at the age of 2. I certainly didn't understand her willingness to continue to avoid me as an adult. I never understood why my stepmother was so violent and spiteful towards me. Despite all I'd gone through, not having my mom in my life, I can contest, was the most difficult thing I've ever had to endure.

When I was just 15 years old, I became pregnant with my first child. This was the first positive shift in my life towards finding my true self. While I understand it now, it wasn't quite as clear to me when I was 16 years old, and a single parent with 2 years of high school to complete. Initially, I was going to put my child up for adoption as I still had 2 years of high school to finish and limited parental support. My stepmother at the time was the one responsible for much of the mental, physical and emotional abuse I endured. Seeing how increasingly spiteful she became towards my daughter, I knew we had to go. I would not live another second with her and put my child through half of what I went through. I remember talking to adoption counselors while I lived in a home for unwed mothers. The more I thought about giving my child up for adoption to ensure she had the best life possible, the more God showed me that this was not His plan for me. I distinctly remember having dreams about my child being abruptly taken away from me. After the third dream, shaken and disturbed, I called my dad and told him I could not give my child away. The feelings of heartache I felt because of my mother's absence is something I never wanted my child to feel. At this point, I knew without a doubt that giving her away was no longer an option. I didn't know how I would finish school and take care of a child. It was at this moment I remember asking God for His help because I had no idea how I would take care of a child and me. I knew deep down to my core that He had given me my daughter for a reason.

When I was 16 years old, I left my parents' home with my 2 month old child. All I had in my possession were the clothes on my back, a diaper bag and a baby in a car seat. We stayed with my half sister and her mom for about 3 months. Due to my sister's mother being unstable and unreliable, I sought shelter with a friend from my grade school. This childhood friend spoke to her mother about my situation, and without hesitation, we moved in. They instantly provided food, clothing and shelter for my child and me. I remember collecting welfare and depending on the state to provide child care services so that I could go to school. During that time, I gave my friend's mother $200.00 a month for allowing my child and me to stay with them. The remainder of the money I used to buy needed items for my child and me. I really called on the Lord to help me, because I didn't know how any of this was going to work out.

In June of 1989, I traveled with my dad, stepmother and siblings to South Carolina for a visit with family. I had no intention of staying and packed just a week worth of clothing for my child and me. Little did I know that a one week trip would end up being a 19 year stay. It took me going to South Carolina to graduate high school on time, as I had unconditional support from my aunt who had cared for me when I was 2 and one of her friends. My aunt's friend cared for my child while I went to school. In the evening, my aunt would pick up my daughter from her friend's house and care for her while I worked to earn the money needed to support us.

When I graduated high school in June of 1990, I applied for a nursing assistant job at a local nursing home. It was in this year that it became mandatory for all persons caring for people in nursing homes and hospitals to have formal training. Earning a certification would allow people to care for those living in nursing homes and seeking care in hospitals. The nursing home I applied to offered to pay for my CNA training and testing. I had always known I wanted to be a nurse, and having the nursing home pay for my initial training to care for others solidified that dream. When I was 8 years old, I remember having a 1week stay at a hospital for a broken arm. I distinctly remember having a compassionate nurse and a somewhat mean nurse. I made sure I told the kind soul that one day I wanted to be a nice nurse like her. Becoming a CNA gave me the foundation and assurance that nursing was what I truly desired to do in life. My career as a nursing assistant was rewarding, and it filled me with gratification. Although I couldn't help myself out of the deep and dark depressed state I was in, I found caring for others filled a missing piece in my heart.

When I first started, I was one of the youngest CNAs working at the nursing home. I was just 18 years old when I met three women who were considerably older than me, as they were nearing retirement age. When I met these 3 women, I was broken, lacked self-esteem and was somewhat of a spitfire. I cursed a lot and was easily frustrated by those I worked with. Almost immediately after I met these ladies, they began encouraging me to go to school and do something more than being CNA. I shared with them some of the things I had been through, and instead of judging me, they challenged me to see my worth, as I couldn't because I was buried in years of pain and hurt.

The nursing home I worked for reimbursed employees going to school for nursing if a C average or better was maintained. Because of my lack of confidence and self-esteem, I declined going to school because I didn't think I was smart enough. I let other people's failures with school dictate my ability to go and succeed. When I did gather up the courage to apply for school, I remember an instructor telling me if I didn't have someone to take care of me financially, I wouldn't be able to complete their nursing program successfully. Despite my desire to become a nurse since I was 8 years old, I walked away from my dream again. When I reached 6 years of being a CNA, I began to doubt I would ever become a nurse. I left the nursing home after six years to work in a fiberglass plant. The company paid double what I made working as a CNA. I used the extra money to pay off unnecessary bills.

After working 3 1/2 years at the fiberglass plant, I soon realized I didn't have the physical stamina, nor the desire, to work production or on an assembly line, removing tubes filled with fiberglass yarn onto respective trucks that were then sent to end finders who cleaned up the product for final processing. During my time working at the fiberglass plant, I had surgery on both of my hands for Carpel Tunnel. I recovered and returned to work. Not long after returning to work, I found myself on light duty as my right rotator cuff was inflamed. Immediately following my light duty rotation, I put in my letter of resignation. I didn't want to endure any more surgeries and I missed caring for people in need. I began working at the local hospital as a patient care tech and applied for school.

In September of 1998, another pivotal moment occurred. My biological mom passed away. I had many mixed emotions regarding her death. I was angry and saddened, as I was hoping to one day obtain enough money to travel and see her. When I received the phone call from my dad, I remember feeling devastated. After returning home from her funeral (having used money loaned to me by a close friend), I remember falling down on my knees and screaming out to God to help me. The pain had become so great to bear after losing my mother, I demanded healing. I asked God why and stated that I was feeling hurt and that I needed His help.

In the year 2000, I provided care to a man suffering with Huntington's disease. One day while I was working, I met a lady who came to visit my patient. During her visit, she asked me if I was I saved. I had no idea what saved meant. I had heard the phrase but didn't fully understand what it was all about. The middle-aged woman went on to explain that it's when you accept the Lord as your savior and forgiver of sins. She went on to say that it's a special prayer that you pray. She asked me if I accepted the Lord as my savior, and I immediately said yes. She prayed the prayer with me and told me that I, too, was now saved. I recall feeling a fuzzy-like feeling after accepting the Lord as my savior. Once I was saved, I was baptized a second time, in 2001, changing my faith from Catholic to Baptist. When I was just 8 years old, I attended a Catholic school and was baptized in the Catholic faith. My exposure to God didn't stop when I was a young child - it went on throughout my entire life.

In 2000, I applied for the LPN nursing program, took the entrance exam and was accepted. It wasn't until I completed the nursing program in 2001 that I began to realize that I was capable of doing anything I put my mind to. I began working as an LPN in an assisted living home and skilled nursing facility. My confidence wasn't where it needed to be and the thought of someone telling me I was a nurse and should know certain things was scary at times. Being a new nurse taught me to seek help if I wasn't sure and to appear confident while I sought the right answer. While I worked as an LPN, I realized the importance of CNAs to nurses. They are our eyes and ears when we can't see. A nurse who listens to her CNAs and reacts with a solution not only builds confidence in himself/herself, but also wins the confidence of the CNAs who care for their patients. It was during my time working as an LPN that I began to realize my worth. It was during this time that I began to realize that people enjoyed working with me and being around me. My presence meant something to me after many years of doubting I meant anything to anyone.

Through all the years of caring for those in need, I always said - and will continue to say - that I am at my best when I am taking care of those in need. I am thankful for my nursing degree, but I'm also thankful for the many challenges. Despite them, I never gave up on my dream. I know, without doubt, that having been shown love from my aunt and uncle at a young tender age is what's compelled me to be loving and kind, especially to those who are vulnerable. I shared my story to say this: it doesn't matter how you start but how you finish.

I share my story not for sympathy, but to encourage others and help those in need, even when they can't help themselves. Hurt, pain and trauma are usually the root causes of crimes that land people in prison or dead. I recall reading self-help books along my journey, which I found immensely helpful. I also read versus from my bible, especially during times of distress. I didn't know exactly what I needed, but I knew I needed something in my life to change if I was going to live out my purpose.

While finishing nursing school a second time, I met my husband, who was also in school pursuing a Bachelor of Social Work. I graduated in May of 2015, and a year later we were married. We made the decision together, after marrying in Las Vegas in April of 2016 that we wanted to someday relocate to Nevada. With careful planning and teamwork, we began our journey in April of 2017. We loaded our personal belongings into a POD to be shipped later and moved out of our 2 bedroom apartment to a 1 bedroom apartment on the east side of Milwaukee. I remember asking God to allow me to live in Wisconsin as an adult, due to my leaving so abruptly at the age of 17. After living back in Wisconsin for 8 years and knowing I would be relocating out of the state soon, I had a desire to live on the east side of Milwaukee. Being on the east side puts you closer to the lake and many fun activities, not to mention my job was within walking distance. We lived in this one bedroom apartment for about 5 months before we began our journey to Las Vegas, Nevada.

When we came to Nevada, we knew we wanted to purchase a home within 1 year. My husband and I began looking at houses at the end of January 2018. When we were getting ready to leave the office after speaking with a sales associate, she remembered that she had a move in ready home similar to the model home we were interested in purchasing. We went to look at the home and it had everything we wanted. My husband wanted the 3 car garage, and I wanted stainless steel appliances. We both wanted the master bedroom and laundry room on the first floor. When we walked into this home, it had all of the above - and then some. Long story short, we moved into our brand new home March 6th, 2018. I share this story because I want others to know and understand that through our faith in God, we can do and become anything our hearts desire. I never in my wildest dreams thought that I would own a home, let alone the kind of home I'm currently living in. Life can seem so unfair at times, but I know and understand that God can't use you if you haven't been through something.

I always told myself if I survive my childhood, which I did, I would have a story to tell. Surviving was half the battle; dealing with the emotional scarring was another. Until I could find my way out of darkness, I consumed much of my time working and helping others. It kept my mind off of my personal problems and filled the void of emptiness I felt in my heart for many years. I'm not saying nursing is the answer for everyone, but, rather, helping others when we can't help ourselves can lead us down a path of success. Processing the hurt and pain and using it for the good of others was my saving grace, along with knowing God and having faith in Him. They say in times of trouble, use God's words to get through. I recall a couple of versus that helped me get through tough times: "I can do all things through Christ who strengthens me" (Philippians 4:13); "No weapons formed against me shall prosper" (Isaiah 54:17); "When my father and mother forsake me, then the Lord will take me up" (Psalm 27:10). I found comfort and strength in knowing that if I believed in God, He would never leave nor forsake me.

Surviving abuse of any kind and using it for the good of others can be done, but many times we find hurt people hurt others. I have wanted to write for a long time now. I also recall reading somewhere, when I inquired about becoming an author, to tell your story at a time when it will impact many. I believe telling my story now will help others choose a different path in life. A path that excludes hurting but helps others. As I stated earlier, with the proper support, we can achieve anything in life we put our mind to. Many times you may feel alone and defeated, but having faith in God can make a world of difference. Having faith in God helps one understand that God can't work without those who accept Him and desire to do good for and by others. Surviving trauma and having the courage to share your story will not only help others, but also help the one who has experienced the trauma. I hope that my story will give hope to those who may be going through similar traumas. When we choose to love and encourage one another, this is when we know God is at work.

Biography

Dawn Bork is a Registered Nurse who specializes in hospice nursing. She has been providing bedside care for 30 years in various capacities. Although this is her first writing, she's looking forward to publishing more books to help those struggling with trauma and abuse. Her goal is to inspire others to find purpose and to succeed in life despite obstacles.

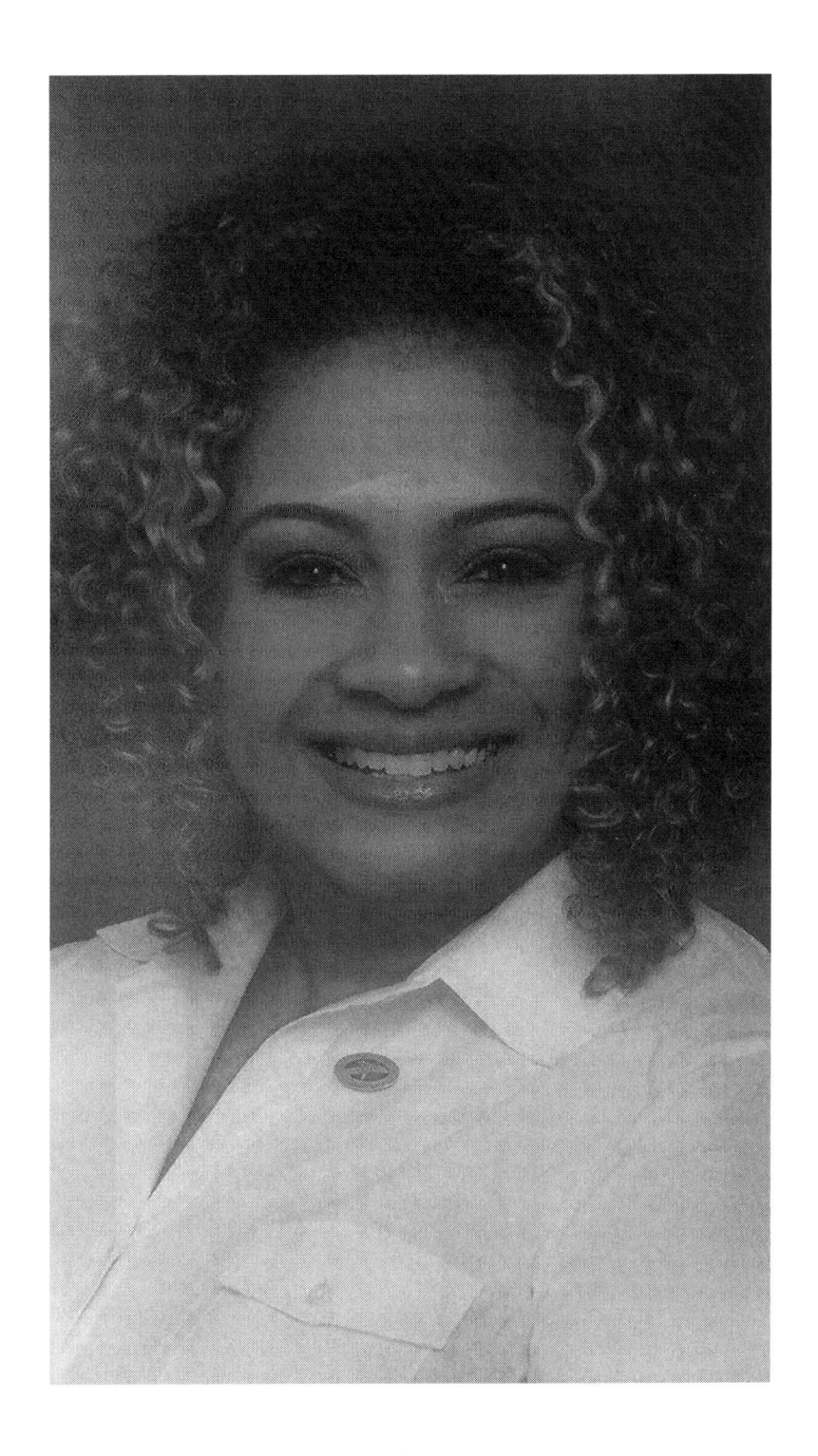

Acknowledgements

I dedicate this chapter to my parents – Elizabeth "Dorothy" Fullard & Oliver Harrod. My Heart and Rock!!! Also, to my siblings – Deborah Gaters; Kenneth Harrod, Sr. and Dawnika Houston. Legacy for my nieces and nephews – Gregory, Juanita, Kenneth, Jr., Justice, KenShawn, Jasmine, Jamera, Jayla & great-nieces and nephews – Jayla, Jameira, Juan, Javon and Morgan. Thanks to family and friends for your support.

Feathers May Fall, But Wings Will Fly

By Charlene Harrod-Owuamana, AAS LPN HBOT WC

It goes without saying that the farther up the climb, the greater the fall. And the bigger the fall is, the worse the consequences will be. Whether you're looking down from the top of a staircase or from the top of a mountain, the danger of falling is always present, but the scale is much different between the two. As far back as I can remember, I've always been scared of heights and equally petrified of falling. I'm not exactly sure where the fear comes from, whether I was born with it or whether it was something I learned early on, but I do know that the fear is palpable and real. Falling is a feeling of complete helplessness, lost ground, lost footing and loss of self. In other words, it's horrifying. You could say that flying is on the other end of the spectrum. Not much different than falling, except perhaps in terms of perspective – because how can you really tell one from the other?

The technical cause for a fear of heights involves proprioception, or the unconscious perception of movement and spatial orientation. Sometimes, being in a anxiety-causing situation - like being high up – can overwhelm the senses and decrease executive function, resulting in a lessening of one's self due to loss of orientation in space. So, you could say that a fear of heights is a result of disconnection from yourself. That disconnection from myself has been the biggest obstacle for me in terms of realizing my true purpose in life, and I believe that the manifestation of this fear in my life has been a critical element in keeping me on the path. I know what it's like to lose sight of my purpose, but I've also experienced many of those small moments that bring me back to it. Those I like to look at as my feathers – delicate, weightless reminders from the angels to focus on the little things and reinvest in self-care.

My childhood was a happy one. As far back as I can remember, I wanted to be a doctor or nurse. I remember one African American nurse, specifically, who worked at the clinic I went to. I always prayed that she would be the nurse to call my name as I sat in the waiting room, and I always let her know this when I saw her. It wasn't often that I saw nurses who looked like me, and seeing her meant so much to me. For as long as I can remember, I would spend my free time at the library, reading all I could get my hands on about nursing. And I can remember how excited my parents would be every year when they would read my Christmas list and see that a doctor's or nurse's bag was front and center. Every year I received one, and I'd always request a new one the following year.

When I was twelve years old, my mom moved my siblings and me out of the projects when she became the caretaker for my grandfather and his sister, my Aunt Clara. This meant moving into a three-story house in West Baltimore, and it was a drastic change for all of us. I remember vividly the heartbreak of leaving my friends. Sure, it was muddled with the knowledge that we were moving up and changing our environment for the better, but it was definitely bittersweet to let go of what was. People tend to think that living in the projects is all bad or that it's shameful and dark, but that's just a one-dimensional view of a very layered existence. Living together in a building with lots of other low-income families brings people together like little else. The relationships we formed with our neighbors were strong and are some of the most beautiful connections of my life that I look back on with great fondness. We didn't have to lock our doors, and there was definitely an unfettered spirit of community present.

But as much good as you can squeeze out of a tough situation, there comes a time when you know it's time to leave. My mom's decision to move us out of the projects literally saved my life. No questions asked. When I look back at my friends who stayed, they are either dead or involved with drugs, and I don't pretend to think that I would have escaped that sort of future had I stayed with them in the projects.

We moved up – higher. Closer to flying or closer to falling, I don't think I was sure. And my fear stayed with me.

My earth shook the night our home burned down. From my room on the top floor, an angel took me out of the window. I don't mean an angel dressed as a firefighter or an instinct to leave through the window that I later referred to as an angel. I mean an actual angel. I know I'd never make my way out of a third story window any other way. My fear of heights was too real. The thing is, no one believed me. They all looked at me like a child making things up. Even my psychiatrist responded with the cold statement that would forever be ingrained in my mind, "There's no such thing as angels." I didn't say a word to her after that.

My mom and youngest brother didn't make it out that night, and I remember waiting for what seemed like an eternity for my other brother and younger sister to be rescued from the flames. Somewhere buried beneath all my grief and sadness was a kernel of something…of knowing that I was saved for some reason, some purpose. I could have just as easily been one of us who didn't make it out. But there I was. It was a feather, something to hold onto.

The cause of the fire was faulty wiring in the refrigerator plug. Imagine that. Here's this appliance set up wrong, not properly wired to do the job it was meant to do. And look at how detrimental that misalignment turned out to be.

What stood out to me in the midst of all my grief was how no one believed me about the angel. I really took this to heart and vowed never to be the kind of person who refuses to believe someone when they tell you something. Not having that acknowledgement led me to develop a brand of empathy that is especially rare. And you would think this would have inspired me onto a path that meant enrolling in pre-med or nursing school, just like I had dreamed of my whole life. Instead, I only got through a year and half before I did a complete three sixty and started studying computers.

Something had stopped me. Like that nagging fear of heights, I had the chance to go up higher, but I panicked and took another route.

I graduated with a degree in computers and spent a handful of years working in that field. At 27 years old, I realized that my life was lacking in a very subtle but potent way. I missed caring for people. The work that I was doing was unfulfilling because it didn't light me up. I recognized that I somehow put myself into a position where I didn't have to do the thing that I was best at. It might've been a way of hiding or of staying safe. There's not much danger of letting your guard down when you work with computers, but there's not that much fulfillment, either (for me, anyway). That's when I decided to go back to school to become a nurse. And it suited me so well. My mom had died overnight in the fire, and now I worked night shifts. It fit together nicely, especially since everyone always referred to me as a "night owl." It was yet another feather on my path, and I was finding my way.

I worked at John Hopkins for many years. Because I worked at an inner-city hospital, I knew that 76% of our population would end up receiving dialysis. Here was another feather. I wanted to give back, and the loudest impact I could make would be by choosing to give back through the National Kidney Foundation. I knew the local Maryland/Delaware branch made a true difference in the lives of patients and their families, so I registered to do a rappel off a twelve-story building to raise money for their cause. That's when I had to face my fear of heights for real. Twelve stories were definitely high and formidable, but I was able to get through it with minimal trouble. Maybe part of that came from the high of being within two days of my fiftieth birthday, and I was feeling fear a little less intensely in that moment. Either way, I rappelled successfully and was thrilled with the accomplishment.

The next year, I wanted to give back through the same charity and registered to rappel again. This year, however, the building had more than doubled in size. This time, we were to repel down a twenty-eight-story building. Now, my fear of heights was really going to be put to the test.

I remember vividly how quiet and peaceful it was at the top of the building looking out at my normally noisy city. From my position near the edge of the building, I saw a man walking toward me. He could see that I was scared, and he was there offering some calm advice before I started my descent, but my conversation with him was totally transformed in my own consciousness. It was like I was having a conversation with God, and He was telling me that He would always be on my side because I heard entirely different words than what that man was actually saying.

He looked at me and said, "Just look into my eyes and focus on me."

What I heard was, "Look into my eyes, my child."

He said, "Just grab this bar and pull yourself up."

I heard, "Reach your arms out to me and pull yourself up."

He said, "Now have a seat, like you're in a chair."

I heard, "Sit back in my arms; I will help you to relax and take you safely to the bottom."

I trusted the voice completely and knew I was safe. Even so, that was the longest five minutes of my entire life. But I did it. I made it to the bottom safely, and I can honestly say that I no longer have a fear of heights. They aren't entirely comfortable for me, but doing anything up high is no longer impossible and doesn't invoke the intense fear that it once did. It now feels like something that I've conquered, and I know that anything is doable, albeit just a little uncomfortable.

You could say that I found myself, and my purpose, that day I rappelled down the twenty-eight-story building. And to be clear, it's not like finding your purpose in life suddenly means that your life becomes easy. The obstacles don't just jump out of your way once you've found a path. The thing that happens when you find your purpose is you now have a lamp with you on your journey. I had faced this fear with God by my side, and I now had a lamp that I could use to light the way. But it wasn't instantly easy.

About two and half years ago, I found myself clinically depressed. I isolated myself from everyone. I wouldn't go out. I wouldn't talk about it. I even abandoned my family by being absent and silent. I felt like I was a failure to them, but I was helpless to do anything about it. At the time, I was working in a methadone clinic, and I'm sure that being in that environment every day wasn't helping with my state of mind.

But then another feather dropped. A young boy came into the clinic and no one there was willing to help him. The instant I looked at him, I saw my younger brother, the one who had passed away all those years ago. I knew unequivocally that I had to help this child, and so that's what I did. And in helping him, I somehow broke out of my funk. Perhaps, in helping him, I was able to release some of the guilt I had about not being able to save my brother. Whether it was guilt or fear, something lifted. I found myself a counselor and made my way out of the darkness.

If it wasn't clear already, it was even clearer now. My main purpose in life was to care for people. And beyond just caring, my goal was to give people that extra special bit of nurturing that is so often missing in healthcare.

It's been more than forty years since I lived in my old neighborhood, but I've gone back to the clinic there. It's here that I'm able to offer something that is so precious to these people, something that is not usually available to them. Because I was raised in the neighborhood, I understand the dynamic like an outsider couldn't, and I know what they need the most has nothing to do with actual medicine or treatment. The people in this neighborhood have never had an advocate. They've never had someone who took the time to explain their healthcare to them. They've never had a provider who looked out for them to make sure they came back for their follow-ups.

That's who I am for them. And because I stood where they once stood, I can give them this support as naturally as if I was talking to my own family and guiding them through the process. I'm able to serve as their advocate and to teach them to be proactive about their health. And I'm there every time they walk through that door.

Currently, I work as a supervisor at this clinic, which is a position that I never actually sought out. My goal was always just to help, not to oversee anyone. However, it's amazing for me to see how supportive everyone is of me in this management role. The staff supports me one hundred percent. And I know that I'm fulfilling my mission, because the patients tell me that if I wasn't here, they wouldn't come in. When I see patients come back for an appointment, it speaks volumes to me because I know how much more likely it was that they wouldn't come back for an appointment. They had to have felt how much I was truly invested in their well-being to actually come back, and I can't imagine a better thank you than to see them back in the clinic.

When patients come back, and tell me that they are glad I'm still here, my heart fills with joy. More than any other time in life, I feel empowered knowing that I am in exactly the right place. It's so humbling to know that my presence helps people every single day. All this support is just another feather confirming that I'm living life exactly as God intended.

I've climbed quite a way since I was that young girl immersed in her nursing books at the library that is no longer standing. And as a girl petrified of heights, I might look at how high I've climbed and be scared for the older me. Scared of messing up, scared of not being enough or scared of being a failure. The young me would be petrified of falling. But the older me has gone through enough to know I'm not falling at all – with every time a patient comes back in, with every bit of jargon that I make easier to understand and with every person that I listen to instead of talk at, I am not falling at all - quite the opposite, actually. The night owl has finally collected enough feathers to fly.

Biography

Charlene Harrod-Owuamana has over 30 years of experience in healthcare. Currently, she is a professional Licensed Practical Nurse with her Associate of Arts Degree and 1st time ambassador & co-author of *We Are Women of Substance*. She's the Founder/CEO of *Nursz's Hive*; hosted her 1st 6-week program at Safe Alternative Foundation for Education, providing mentorship for youth in her city. She is the former president and Founder of *Black Nurses Rock Baltimore*, Maryland chapter, where she changed lives by educating the community in which she served. At the Maryland Board of Nursing, she's on the advisory committee for CNAs/GNAs and assists with the approval of CNA/GNA programs. She is an advocate for LGBTQ community and a speaker for two years at "Baltimore in Conversation". She's very active in the community given back to the youth; by participating in Vivien T. Thomas Medical Arts Academy Nursing Assistance Program – pinning ceremony in 2017. Charlene has a true passion for training and sharing her expertise within the healthcare systems. She's been a pediatric nurse for over 18 years and over 30 years in the Healthcare System. Focusing on continuing her studies in Healthcare Administration and the Nursing field. She has been given the title of "Super Nurse" & "Nurseologist; because of her ability to share her knowledge and creative ideas with others. She will leave you empowered and inspired with her community evolvement. She has a goal to become a professional speaker and impact live in her city and around the country. She returned to her old neighborhood to provide excellent nursing care to West Baltimore. She also has been elected "Employee of the Month" twice in one year.

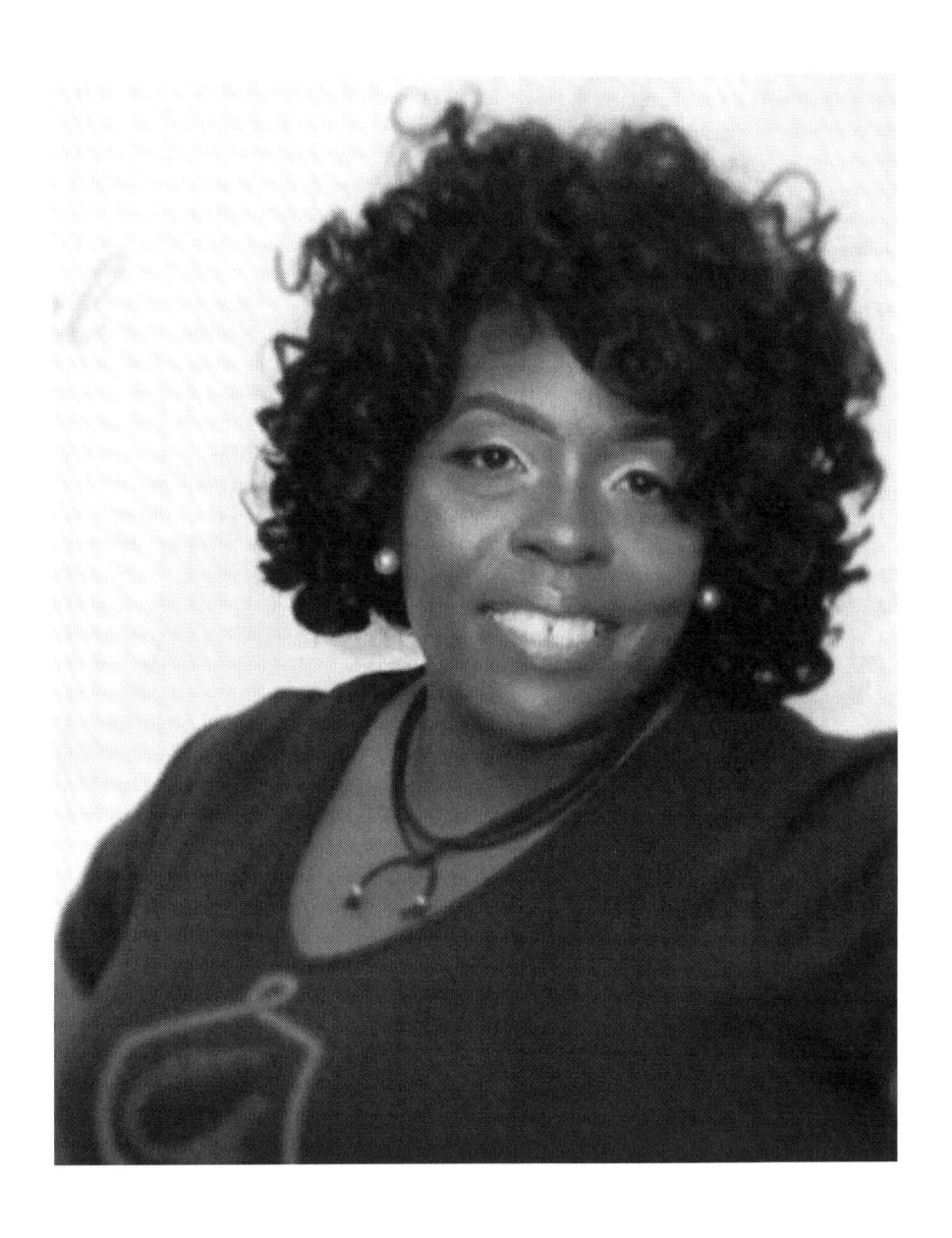

Acknowledgements

I am humbled and eternally grateful to my Lord and Savior, Jesus Christ, for His constant Grace and Mercy, for always walking with me and sometimes carrying me through life's journey. I know that I could do nothing without Him, but with Him, I can do ALL things.

I would like to dedicate this book to my handsome sons, DeJai J. Mitchell and Alphie D. Guillory, Jr. Thank you for your unconditional love and support, and for being patient with me while I strived to give you both the best. I honestly don't know who I would be without you both. You are my PURPOSE! I love y'all!!

And lastly, to my parents, Big Jell (Grandma Jellybean), and my family who have been in my corner from the beginning. Special thanks to Aunt B, Aunt Peb, and Uncle Marq - my cheering squad. To each person who has influenced and touched my life in some way throughout the years, I say "thank you!"

Onissa

"All people are NOT soldiers and just because they have the desire doesn't mean they are qualified." (Pastor Billy Weaver)

CHOZEN
Discovering Purpose in Life and in Nursing

By Onissa S. Mitchell, MSN, RN, APRN, FNP-C

"For many are called, but few are chosen." Matt 22:14

Have you ever wondered what your purpose in life is? Why you are truly here? Why you do the things you do or act the way you act? Why you are determined to succeed or why you don't allow anything or anyone to stop you from reaching your goals? Are you thirsty or hungry for something more but just can't seem to pinpoint why you feel this way? Why do you dream so big? These types of questions are raised both consciously and subconsciously within each of us. Some choose to ignore them while others seek out answers, trying to identify their driving force.

As we go through life, we grow and develop. We change. We go through ups and downs, trials and tribulations, whether these experiences are good, bad, ugly or indifferent. Within the storms and the chaos, we find strength, set goals, have dreams and find something greater that drives us. What drives you?

Purpose

What is the meaning of purpose? Purpose has been defined as doing something with determination; a function, role or use. It is the reason for which anything is done, created or exists. Purpose is having an aim or intention in mind. It's something for which you strive. Biblically, purpose is showing reverence to God; to fear and obey Him. So, I ask, have you found your purpose, or you do you know what your purpose is? Is your purpose aligned with God's will? What are your goals, aspirations…YOUR PURPOSE?

Background

To fully understand what I'm building, you have to understand my foundation. I was born in a small east Texas town where everybody was familiar with everybody's family. As a matter of fact, all the families in my town had some type of "-ship:" friendship, kinship, or personal, business, or romantic relationship. Yes, they were all connected in some way and we took pride in these connections. I guess you can say our small town was more of a "village." Most families in my "village" ensured that the children didn't misbehave or step out of line while also showing compassion and kindness to everyone. However, if someone did, in fact, display inappropriate behavior, well, let's just say he/she was not only disciplined by his/her immediate family, but also by the adult that witnessed the wrongdoing. People possessed mutual respect for each other and were committed to these "-ships." The age-old saying that "it takes a village to raise a child" was at its core.

We lived a simple life without the burden of lots of material possessions. We had each other, our basic needs, and most importantly, love. My parents were young – still in school - when my brother and I were born, so you can only imagine their struggles. They were faced with trying to complete high school, work and raise two children all while dealing with the stigma associated with teenage parenting. After high school, my mother was forced to put her life, hopes and dreams of becoming a nurse on hold to ensure the two lives she brought into this world were covered. She worked her butt off to make sure we were cared for. My father left our small town to pursue his education and career goals. He called frequently and visited during college breaks as well as holidays, but maintaining a long-distance relationship took its toll. Unfortunately, he had to sacrifice his desire to be available for his family to ensure he was able to provide in the future. I'm sure there were times he wanted to be a more present figure in our lives; however, he was seeking answers and trying to find his own purpose. As he found his way and became more financially stable, he was able to be somewhat more available. He would come to our sporting events and other school events as much as he could, but living so far away didn't allow him to be as present as we needed. He did at least try. You see, he built his life in the city, and traveling in excess of four hours one-way can get a little expensive and take a toll on a person, to say the least. My parents did their best to instill good values and morals in us. We knew they loved us and that was good enough.

School Days

Education had always been important to my parents, but when you're 4 years old, how would you know that? Well, somehow it was ingrained within my subconscious at birth, or I was just being dramatic. You may laugh, but I'm so serious. I was determined to go to school even though I was too young for kindergarten. Heck, my brother was going so why couldn't I go? You must understand that my brother is and has always been my best friend. If you saw him, you were going to see me, and if you didn't, I wasn't far behind. I remember throwing such a big temper-tantrum that the principal at my brother's school found a way to allow me to enter school an entire year early. Her willingness to look pass my age - even though I was being a little stinker - gave me the opportunity to go to school, which was only the beginning of my educational pursuits.

My desire to be in that school with my brother and mimic his every move was the first display of the determination that lived within me. Nobody recognized it at the time, but in hindsight, I believe that was the initial glimpse into my developing character. During my school-age years, I excelled academically. Work ethics were developed that surpassed most children in my age group. While others were playing and partying with their friends, I was studying most of the time. I'm not saying that I never attended events with my friends, but if there were assignments that were not completed, I was home getting them done. It appeared as though knowledge was a driving force; an unquenchable thirst. Learning gave me joy. I was nerdy, indeed, but I was also an athlete. I participated in every sport I could play. I was good at some of them while not so much at others. People seemed to like me for the most part as I was a social butterfly: outgoing, friendly, intelligent, tomboyish and athletic; yep, that was me. I didn't really have to deal with bullying except if I was stepping in to help someone who was being bullied. My teachers loved me as I didn't give them any problems, did my work and acted accordingly.

The Transition

College was always a goal and not going wasn't really an option for me. As I said before, education was and still is very important to my parents, especially my mother. Remember, my father was able to further his education, but my mother sacrificed hers for us. She didn't get the opportunity to pursue her educational dreams; therefore, it was imperative that her children did.

In my third year of college, I became pregnant by my high-school sweetheart. Here I was, 20 years old, trying to finish what my mother didn't...and pregnant. With disbelief, I took 3 additional pregnancy tests to confirm this to be true. Depression and devastation set in with abortion at the forefront of my mind. My parents were going to be so disappointed, but my mother was going to kill me. I never thought I would get pregnant at this age, especially not while I was in college. How was I going to explain this to them? How will they respond? I saw my entire life flash before my eyes and my dreams of having a college degree were shattered.

I called my best friend and her first question was "what do you want to do?" You would have to know my best friend to understand that she was going to support my decision regardless. I told her that I wasn't prepared financially or emotionally to have this baby. Plus, my high-school sweetheart was no longer mine. I told her, "I need to get an abortion." My best friend paused for a second and then said, "I will send you the money." Despite having the means, my heart and conscious wouldn't allow me to harm this baby. I finally gained enough courage to tell my family and surprisingly they were okay. Yes, they were disappointed, but they provided reassurance and support.

Faith Test

The pregnancy and birth were plagued with complications and my son was born at 25-weeks gestation with breech presentation. He was very small, weighing 1 lb. 11.9 oz. We spent the next 3 months living in the Neonatal Intensive Care unit. I was an emotional basket case during this time as I wasn't sure if he was going to live. The doctors and nurses were very supportive but honest with me about his prognosis. His potential for normalcy was not good, and though I was scared, I was also hopeful. Sleepless nights became my norm as I was worried about his future and mine. I became overwhelmed and wanted to give up until I heard God's voice say, "Trust Me." How could I? My son is so small and it's possible that he will be medically fragile. What exactly does that mean?

Before you can understand my breakthrough, you must first know my been-through. The next 1 to 2 years were filled with peaks and valleys. I went back and obtained that degree, moved to Dallas and started a new life with my son, but he wasn't reaching his development milestones. Delays were expected due to his prematurity, but he should have been making some progress by now. He was still having difficulty sitting up without assistance, holding his head up, rolling over and had yet to start vocalizing (making sounds) at almost 2 years old. He was able to smile, frown and cry but no crawling, walking or talking. Something was not right. My suspicions were confirmed when my sweet, happy boy was diagnosed with Cerebral Palsy. I was told that he might not live past the age of 5 and even if he did, he would never be able to live independently. How was a 22-year-old supposed to process and respond to this? With tears in the wells of my eyes, I looked at the doctor, saying, "You don't have the final say!" I had no idea what this diagnosis was, nor what kind of impact this would have on our lives. "Lord, how am I supposed to do this?" I asked with fear and pain in my heart. "Trust Me," the Lord whispered back. Hopeless, devastated, angry and defeated was only part of what I felt. Here was this beautiful, innocent little boy with a smile that lit up the world and he was confined to a body that didn't work. He didn't deserve that! I didn't deserve to be "stuck" with this type of burden. What did he do to deserve this? What did I do?

After the initial shock of this new discovery, I decided to fight. I flashed back to watching him in that incubator for 3 months, fighting for his life; fighting because I asked him to. So, now it's my turn; I will fight for him. As I gazed into those big brown eyes, I wiped my tears and said, "Are you ready, Son? I won't quit until you quit!" He gave me the biggest smile that I'd ever seen, as if he was saying "Let's get it done, Momma." From that day until this one, we fight daily and neither of us has any desire to quit.

New Addition

In February 2001, my 2nd son was born. He was a healthy baby with no deficits or issues. He reached every milestone as expected and brought so much joy into our lives. His father and I were engaged and in the process of buying a house, so we should be good, right? Wrong!!! He sold me a dream and I was so blinded by love that I believed it. He made me believe that we were going to build a life together and live happily ever after. Unfortunately, that was far from the truth. After being made aware that this young man was not totally committed to our family, nor was he interested in being a father to a special needs child, I choose to vacate the relationship. A single parent again, but this time, there were 2.

Purpose Born

Busted, disgusted and angry, yet determined to provide my sons with the best life I could, I returned to school. I wasn't sure what I wanted to pursue, but I had to do something. I now had a purpose and reason to never quit. In my mind, I was placed here for my sons and I would do whatever it took to fulfill that purpose. There were many trials and tribulations we endured in pursuit of happiness. From my oldest son's near-death experience at age 4, to his multiple hospitalizations and surgeries, court dates and custody battles for my youngest son, to broken relationships, including a marriage that ended with divorce, section 8 housing and government assistance, we endured it all. I did what was necessary to ensure my children's needs were met and continued to fight for them both.

You see, before God reveals your ultimate purpose, He will take you through a period of preparation to ensure that you would be willing to own it, accept it and believe it as He truly intends you to do. He will make sure that you are mature enough to handle the greatness that He will bring forth through your purpose.

Pressing on toward the mark was what I continued to strive for. Armed with the strength of God and love of my children, I went on to gain my certification as a Nurse's Aide. I worked hard at the local nursing home, caring for the elderly. Some were physically able to care for themselves while others required total care. I would feed, bathe and groom the residents and then come home to care for my own special patient. My grandmother was so proud that I did not give up or succumb to society's view of what I could accomplish as a young, unwed mother of 2 with one being special. But she saw more. "You gone make a nurse after while," she said. I didn't see this as my path, but I guess God was using her as the messenger to reveal this next step He had for me.

Purpose Unfolding

Driven by my perceived purpose, I continued to work and found much satisfaction in caring for others. It brought a sense of peace and enjoyment that was unexplainable. I looked forward to going to work and spending time with my patients, but financially, this would not sustain my family. Again, I turned back to education. That unquenchable thirst continued to be a driving force for my future, and it still burned strong in my soul. I enrolled in nursing school. I was focused and determined, but I still had to maintain my household while I was on this journey. I worked 2 part-time jobs at night and on weekends, all while attending classes during the day. Studying became something we did as a family, as I had to creatively incorporate my time with the boys into my school work. They didn't get the normal bedtime stories, they learned about anatomy and physiology while they drifted off to sleep, listening to me read to them aloud. You may laugh, but I was serious about providing for them and fulfilling this assignment that God gave me. May 2005, assignment completed. I did it!

Grandma was again proud but had another message, "You gone make a doctor after while." There she goes with that foolish again, right? I surely didn't want to hear that. I had already had too many sleepless nights, missed or reduced time with my boys, stress and anxiety, but God's word never returns void. In August 2013, I completed my Master of Science in Nursing and became a Family Nurse Practitioner. My grandmother passed away in 2015. I remember having to constantly remind her prior to her death that I was not a doctor, and she would say to me, "You're my doctor." It brings me peace to know that, in her eyes, I had accomplished becoming "her doctor." It all was worth it!

Hindsight is 20/20

Let me enlighten you for a moment, just in case you have yet to figure this out: I was CHOZEN by God to be a caregiver. This didn't become evident to me until I began analyzing my past and recognized how effortless it had been for me to show compassion, kindness and patience to others. When I realized that I truly enjoyed providing care for those who were unable to care for themselves, it was clear what my true purpose was. I've cared for something or someone for as long as I can remember. My first dog at 4 years old and the elderly clients that I helped my grandmother with at age 12 were just God's way of preparing me to be a lifetime caregiver for my special-needs child and a great mother for my other son. Did I know this when I was going through all the hell I went through? No! Would I be able to fight relentlessly for my children had I not walked the road I did? Probably not. If I had known I would face the chaos I did, I would not have made the choices I made. I probably would have had that abortion or put my oldest son in a home when my other son's father decided he wasn't able to deal. I probably would have quit years ago, especially with all the failed relationships (including a marriage), financial issues, headaches, heartaches and emotional rollercoasters I've endured over the years, not to mention watching my oldest son suffer multiple health issues and my youngest son move away to live with his father 4 or 5 years ago. Now that almost took me out and caused some mental and emotional pain for both my oldest son and me! I almost threw in the towel as I felt like a complete failure and that I let God and my children down (but that's a story for another day). Despite my own personal feelings about him leaving, my son and I have been able to maintain a strong relationship and have an unbreakable bond. Ensuring that he knows that I will always be available in spite of his decision to leave has been important to me. My boys are and will always be inseparable and their relationship remains remarkable. They are best friends. The youngest is truly his brother's keeper, and it shows. Through the adversity, social stigmas, self-doubt, self-condemnation, trials and tribulations, we've managed to continue standing. My family still stands.

Lessons/Words of Wisdom

Life has been the best teacher and I'm sure there are plenty of other lessons that I have yet to learn. So far, here are just a few:

…...God doesn't let you and nobody else see everything He's doing in your life and He will not allow everyone to go with you to your purpose. Eagles fly alone.

As my sons and I continue our journey, I have learned and continue to be reminded to

….. Trust God and His plan. He will order you steps despite your own apprehension and self-doubt.

…...God does not always reveal your purpose in its entirety at one time. He must make sure that you are ready to receive your purpose and that you are adequately prepared to act on it.

…...You have to be a willing spirit to receive His blessings.

…...Stay focused despite life's distractions.

…...Love like you've never been hurt.

…...Don't seek validation from invalid people because they are not qualified to evaluate your true value!

…...Don't be afraid to walk away from people, including family, places or things that are not supporting your dreams and elevating your purpose. If the person or situation is not helping you, then it's hindering you

……Never dim your light because someone else can't handle your shine. Simply hand him/her some sunglasses and shine brighter.

……Don't worry about other people's opinions about your decisions, because what others think about you is none of your business.

……Make yourself proud, be a good representative of your ancestors and, most importantly. TRUST GOD AND HIS PLAN!!!

Walking in Your Purpose/Closing

As time passes, you will find that you may have more than one purpose; however, you must wait for God to reveal them to you. Each day brings about new challenges, but it also brings new opportunities. New chances to be better than you were yesterday and grow into who God has ordained you to be. You will discover, when you are walking in your purpose, there is peace. Work doesn't feel like work, tasks required of you are effortless and you find joy in the process. You strive to be a blessing to others and make their lives better. Yes, you will always encounter people and situations that will make you question your purpose, but in those times, remember your WHY - why you embarked on this path in the beginning and where you are looking forward to going. Remember what you are trying to accomplish. Negative circumstances and people will test your faith, friends will abandon you and family will not support you. Will you allow it to make you bitter or better? There will be times when you will have to walk alone and times when God allows others to be part of your journey towards your purpose. Remember where you started from, take pride in what you have already overcome and believe in where you are going. Realize that everything that you go through is part of God's process to grow and develop you into your purpose. And most all, never forget, you have been CHOZEN!!

Biography

Onissa S. Mitchell is a single mother of two handsome young men, one of which was born with Cerebral Palsy. She began her career as a Certified Nurse Assistant in 2002-2003 and went on to obtain her Bachelor of Science in Nursing in May 2005. After working in various areas of patient care, she continued her educational endeavors and became a Family Nurse Practitioner. In this role, she has been *providing family-centered healthcare to patients of all ages since August 2013*. Onissa is a strong, patient advocate and uses a holistic approach ensuring that all aspects of wellness are addressed. Her philosophy is and will always be to treat people as you want to be treated and find beauty in everything. Onissa's positive attitude and confidence in the spirit of people has allowed her to be a light in the darkness of her patients and to those who have the privilege of knowing her.

She is the Owner/CEO of Healing Hearts CPR where she ensures her clients are equipped with the knowledge and life-saving skills required to perform high-quality Basic Life Support, CPR, and First Aid. She is also the Owner/CEO of East Texas Drug and DNA Testing where she is a certified collector and Breathe-Alcohol Technician. She uses her expertise to ensure the workplace of her clients remain drug and alcohol-free.

In her spare time, Onissa can be found traveling and enjoying life with her family. She can also be found mentoring nursing students and graduate nurses pursuing their nurse practitioner degree, as well as participating in activities that bring awareness to diseases like heart disease, stroke, autism, and cerebral palsy. Onissa is an active member of the national organization Black Nurses Rock, American Association of Nurse Practitioners, and a proud member of St. Louis Baptist Church in Tyler, Texas.

To contact the author:

FB: https://www.facebook.com/onissa.mitchell

IG: https://www.instagram.com/godschozenfnp

Email: onissamitchell@gmail.com

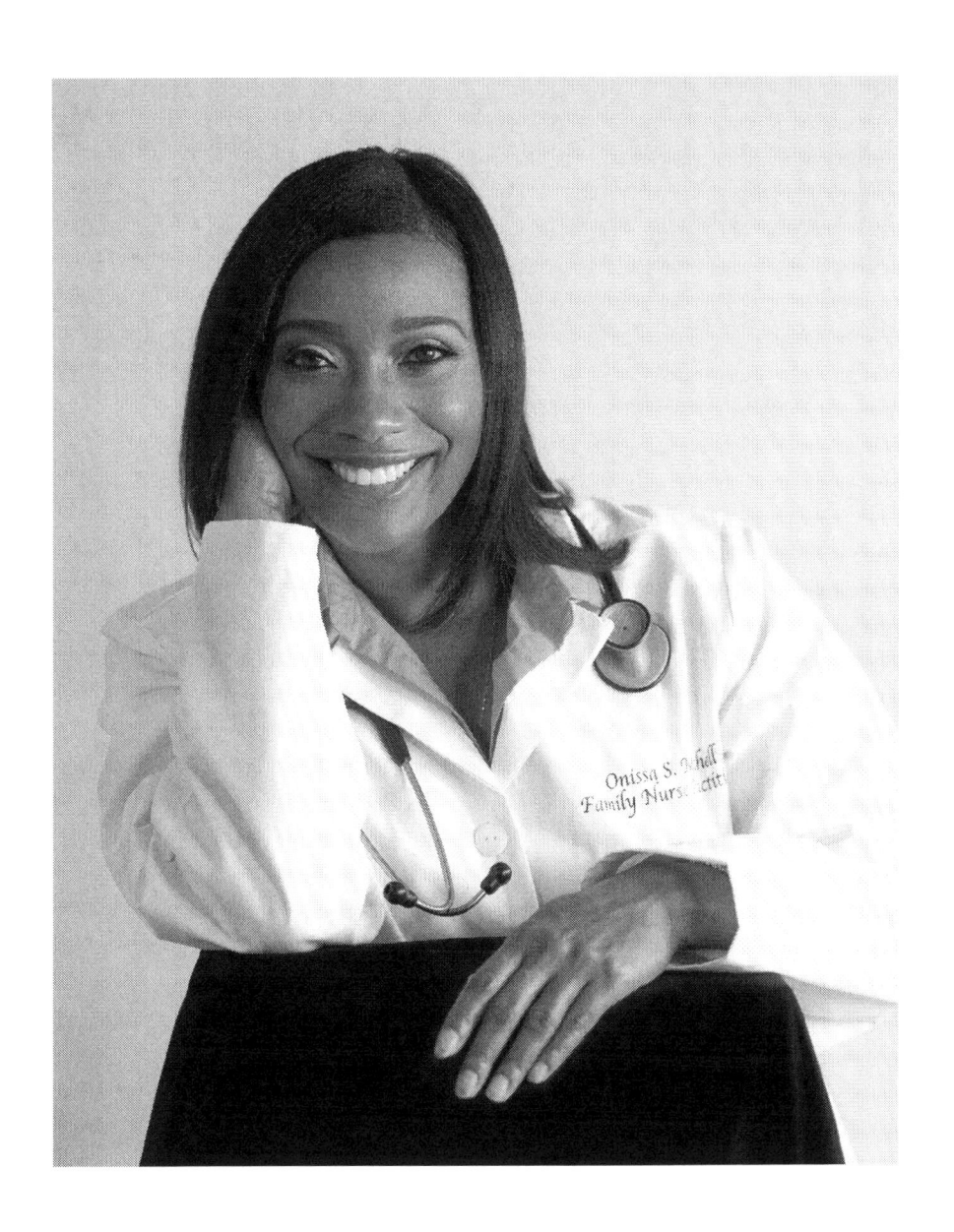

Dark Beginnings Don't Have to Mean Dark Endings
Women on Purpose

By Lola Olarunfemi

"Thieves don't raid houses where there is no treasure."
~ Unknown

I landed in this world with a thump like the day's mail lands in the mailbox - the kind of mail that is all bills and warning notices, not birthday cards and packages. My dad was already gone. He had left my mother when she was eight months pregnant with me. And my mother handed me off as well, first to my grandmother and then, more permanently, to my aunt, by the time I was three years old.

My aunt and her husband raised me, alongside their two sons, but I was never a part of the family. She used tell my cousins that I had a strange spirit; that there was a bad force in me. She also believed that girls and boys should be raised differently. That was why I was the one always doing the laundry, scraping the dishes and prepping the chickens after they were butchered. Really the difference between how they raised the boys and how they raised me seemed to be more like the difference between how you treat your child and how you treat a slave. I didn't say much about it. I did the chores that were expected of me and kept my head down.

Worse than the chores was the abuse. Both my aunt and her husband both verbally and physically abused me. My aunt's mantra to me was, "You're not gonna amount to anything."

I heard that sentiment phrased all sorts of ways, but the meaning was always plain. I was a worthless burden, headed nowhere. I could never quite understand why this blood relative of mine had such a vivid distaste for me. As much as it hurt, all I could do was try my best not to let it get to me.

They paid for my schooling, but I paid for it all the same because the cost was just their green light to do whatever they wanted to me. "We pay your tuition, so that means we can treat you however we want," said my aunt's husband on many occasions. And when they'd have friends over, I'd shake in fear, because I knew those friends would find their way to me. They'd do what they wanted to me in whatever dark room they could find. They'd tell me I couldn't tell anyone or they'd kill me. And all I could do was believe them, and let it happen. There was no one on my side in the house to tell, anyway.

Often I wondered where my mother was, and why she hadn't shown up to take me back. She and my aunt still talked at this point, so my aunt knew where she was living. She simply chose to keep that from me. I learned much later that the image she painted of what my life was like was much different than reality, and from those happy and hopeful descriptions, my mother assumed I was doing well. To her, I was simply one less thing she needed to worry about. If I was doing fine, that was good enough for her.

My aunt and her husband drowned me in chores. I was responsible for nearly everything to keep the house running. I did the laundry, washed the dishes and even washed the cars, which based on my aunt's rationale, I'd have thought would've been a task for the boys, but that fell to me, too. The discrepancy between what I was responsible for and what my cousins were responsible for was a gigantic chasm. They got to be kids, playing and focusing on their schoolwork, while I slaved away doing everything for the house. If I wanted to get my schoolwork done, I had to carve out a few hours in the middle of the night to do it.

There was one occasion where my aunt needed three chickens prepped. She gave me two to do, and my cousin was supposed to take care of the other one. I prepped mine as I always did, and went to bed. Later than night, I was sound asleep and abruptly awoken when she poured a bucket of ice water on my head. Confused and dazed from sleep, I asked what was going on. She yelled at me for leaving a chicken undone in the kitchen. I explained that I prepped my chickens and it had to be my cousin's that was still there, but she didn't care. She took all my clothes and my things for school, which was a common reaction for them when they were angry with me. I had to walk barefoot to school the next day because I knew there was a test that I couldn't miss. I refused to let something so silly as a chicken prevent me from taking my exam.

And as I got older, the abuse and neglect increased. By the time I was thirteen years, old, I was getting hit and slapped on a daily basis. I always was very religious, so once the abuse became that regular, I reached out to God and asked Him daily, "What did I do wrong?"

I begged Him to speak to me, to guide me, to give me some peace of mind. I was always a big reader so I wasn't surprised when His answer to me came in one of the books I was reading. I don't remember the exact quote or book, but the message was clear: "Thieves don't raid houses where there are no treasures. "

That had to be it. This was the only explanation for their unprovoked brutality towards me, and this sentiment became my guiding light. I held on to this idea so tightly. I made it my truth because it was the only thing that made sense. I never asked for the abuse. I never did anything that warranted it. In fact, I did the opposite, trying to be as pleasant and unobtrusive in the house as possible. I studied hard and did my schoolwork religiously. The only thing that made a shred of sense and brought me any comfort was that I was being attacked not because I was worthless but because I wasn't. No one raids a house unless it has something valuable inside. That's how I knew I had to persist. I wasn't being persecuted because I was bad, but because I was good. What a revelation. These people were trying to pilfer that goodness and take it from me. I knew then that I couldn't let that happen; that I had to go on, that I did indeed, have a purpose and something to live for.

Knowing that I had a reason to persist didn't make anything easier. It simply gave me a goal. I still had a slew of obstacles that continued to litter my path. One time, I went to school without washing the dishes, and my aunt's husband smashed my glasses right in my face. The shards of glass shattered all over my eyes, and I nearly went blind from it, but that was what I deserved for leaving the dishes. There wasn't any remorse or even an apology.

As I got older, my aunt's husband's abuse seemed to take on a sexual edge. He never did anything outright, but sometimes he'd come into the bathroom when I was showering, and he'd forbid any social contact with the boys at my school. If he did witness any interaction with a boy, I would pay handsomely. One time he saw me talking to a boy in the library. That night, he ripped my clothes from me and locked me outside. I only had just enough clothes to get by - about three shirts, three skirts and one pair of shoes. I'd have even less after his angry rages, and I'd have to go school in whatever I had leftover.

At one point, he adopted me. You might imagine that an adoption would be a happy occasion for a kid, especially since my mother hadn't ever resurfaced to collect me, but this was not an adoption of love. This adoption was done in the spirit of disownment. He took my name from me, my identity and replaced it with his name. He said, "This is your last name now. If you deny it, I will curse you and you'll die." He had all the records changed so that there was no trace of the old me left. It was like he bought me through my tuition like a used car, and now he was putting his vanity plate on me.

I felt so helpless. I had nowhere to run. I wanted to leave more than anything, but where could I go? Plus, if I left, I had no way of paying my tuition on my own and nowhere to live. I was forced into obedience, and both he and my aunt knew exactly what they were doing. They both worked at the university I attended. My aunt was a librarian, and her husband was a professor. They both did a great job of living this dual life, putting on a pleasant and refined face to the students they interacted with while treating me like trash behind closed doors.

The abuse was regular and daily, but one day went especially sour. My "dad," which is what I called my aunt's husband, got extra violent with me. He punched me hard, and I tried to run away, but I ran into the handle of a door and fractured my jaw. I fell to the ground in pain, and he came after me with a wooden plank. I curled up into the fetal position, but my leg must've been exposed because he brought the plank down hard on my knee. He tore my clothes and took them; he took my shoes. My knee was throbbing and swollen, but I also knew that I had an important test the next day. I could hear the laughter and see the shadows of my cousins going about their night in their respective rooms while I hunkered outside in my underwear scared and afraid. I had to jump the fence and simply wait it out as usual. I didn't eat that night or the next morning and walked fourteen kilometers or more, barefoot. I made it to an office where I begged the woman there for some money to take the bus the rest of the way. She gave me enough money for the bus and a pair of flip flops. I wore another woman's skirt and flimsy sweater as a top, but I made it to school, and I took my test.

I don't know how I passed the test that day, but somehow I did. It wasn't until after the test that I passed out. The stress and the lack of food had finally taken its toll. My friends took me to health services on campus, where the doctor gave me an X-ray for my jaw, a balm for the bruises and some medication to take care of the pain. He asked if I had been in a fight, and I said I hadn't. I told him I was beaten. With a sudden understanding of what was going on, he told me I needed to take a break from that house. For the next three days, I stayed with friends while I healed.

When I finally returned to that house, I showed up with an entirely different mentality and a game plan. I confronted my "dad" and told him that I had stayed away because of what he had done. I said that he could either let me live there peacefully or I'd let the truth come out. The doctor at the clinic made sure I knew that I could come back if anything happened again, so I could tell this man with confidence that he couldn't hurt me anymore. If it happened again, I was welcome to come back to the clinic, if I needed to. I confronted my aunt as well. She asked me why I was back. I countered by asking why she hadn't tried to find me if she knew I was missing. But she just called me a wicked woman and wrote off my disappearance with a wave of her hand. There was no remorse or worry in her words.

I suspect someone in the clinic around that time saw what had happened to me and must've also known where my mother was living and contacted her. Not long after that incident, my biological mother showed up in class one day with my other siblings in tow. I was amazed. She had finally come for me after all these years of wishing. As she tried to get me to come with her, my aunt and her husband claimed that my mother was trying to kidnap me. They pretended they didn't know who she was and started to fight her legally. But luckily my mother had all the proof. She had my birth certificate and confronted her sister with it. I finally got the news from the Dean that my aunt's husband would lose his job. The light seemed to be trickling in.

I had maintained a friendship with the doctor who treated me at Health Services the day my jaw was fractured. Eventually, our relationship developed into something more. Slowly I started feeling comfortable enough to reveal things about myself to him; I began to trust him with my story. He got a job abroad while I was finishing up an internship in my fourth year of school, and he asked if I wanted to join him abroad. I could finish my studies closer to him or join him after I was finished. Either way, I had a plan and a future. I could've stayed and tried to get justice for myself and all those years of torment, but I felt that it was in my best interest to simply walk away and put those years behind me. After all, it wasn't really my place to do the judging. I believed that justice would come from God. So, we got married and moved abroad.

I tried inviting my aunt to the wedding. Her reply was only, "Are you pregnant?" I didn't take the bait. I simply responded that it was a simple invitation. I wasn't here to start trouble. She called me a witch and that was that.

I also was able to track down my biological dad and invited him to the wedding, even though I wasn't quite sure how I felt about it. My fiancé told me to give him a chance and let him be there. He passed away not long after that, and I'm glad that I did give him that chance. I've forgiven both him and my biological mom. I don't quite understand their choices, but I've forgiven them anyway. I currently give my mom a monthly stipend and try to be present in her life, but there's still a lot of hurt there. I don't judge her, but every now and then I feel that pain resurface. I simply don't let it rule me.

My entire childhood and young adult life were incredibly bleak and dark. Looking back, sometimes I'm not sure how I made it through all those shades of abuse and torture. What I do know is that it's no accident that I'm here today, living the life that I'm living. I didn't just happen to make it out of my situation - I made my way out. I am a woman ON purpose. I have so much love to share with the world. The bits of light that led me to where I stand today were tiny and they flickered, so that sometimes it was hard to know they were still there. But I believed and trusted in God. And I kept my mantra close to me. No one raids a house where there are no treasures. If I could hold onto that, then I could believe that there was something worth treasuring in me. I know that I was blessed with good friends and that I was gifted when it came to my studies, and for me, those were shreds of light. I saw as a gift the fact that school came so naturally to me. You can't choose your circumstances, but God equipped me with this great tool, this ability to learn. I started life in a hole, but He gave me a ladder, and there was no way I'd squander that gift.

By no means was any of it easy. For decades, the thing I wanted most in the world was a simple hug, or a kind word that never came from the people closest to me. I'd cry alone, I'd cry in the rain and I'd tell God what I felt on those days. And I just knew, in my gut, that one day it would end. One day, I'd get myself out. If my aunt and her husband were going to use my tuition as an excuse to mistreat me, than I was going to use that degree to leave them for good. So, I worked hard. I worked hard because my life depended on it. Those times when I was bruised and my clothes were ripped, I made sure I went to school anyway. If I didn't, I'd be letting my aunt and her husband win. That's what they wanted. They wanted to see me fail. They wanted me to try to leave and come crawling back because I couldn't get by without them. But all that only made me stronger and more motivated to change my surroundings.

Originally, I got my degree in Real Estate and Asset Management, but it didn't take long for me to realize that my true passion was helping others. So, I went back to school for nursing, and now my career allows me to make a difference in people's lives every day. That part of me that was never cared for or taken care of gets to reach out and help others regularly. And when I see a patient smile, or when I can see that I provided some semblance of comfort or guidance to a person in need, I know that my purpose is real.

Once I did confront my mom about the past, and I asked her a simple question. I asked, "Do you know what it feels like to not have a home?" She looked at me with her cola colored eyes that are strikingly similar to my own, and she said nothing. She just stared back at me. Maybe that silence was the best that she could do in that moment. Maybe she understood, and there was no way she could acknowledge the deep pain that she set me into and silence was her only choice. Or maybe she couldn't grasp it at all. I don't know. What I do know is that not having a home makes you feel like a nobody. There's no single place in the world where a door is always open to you. You don't have a safe space where you know you can always retreat and find comfort. But that silence that she gave me is the spark where my purpose begins. That void and emptiness that I received is the exact void that I am meant to fill in others. Because I persisted, I now stand in shoes that no one can take from me, and I can give to others the exact thing that I never received. I can choose to end the cycle of neglect, and instead create and give something beautiful. I don't have to share hate because hate is what I got. The hurt and the pain stop with me. I get to ensure that the lost and the lonely souls I encounter on my path know that my door is always open to them.

There's a treasure here in me, and my purpose is to share that light and love with the world.

Biography

Lola Olarunfemi is am a Registered Nurse, Faculty / Clinical Instructor, Legal Nurse Consultant, Author and Entrepreneur. She has worked in both US and Canada. She is currently a faculty member at the University of Northern British Columbia . She hold a Bachelors and Masters in Nursing. She also has a Bachelors degree in Real Estate and Asset Management prior to becoming a Nurse.

She has experience in Med/ surg, Telemetry, Psychiatry/ Behavioral Health, Home Health, Long- term Care and Nursing Education.

She proudly serves as the CEO of Lola Health Consulting -a Legal Nurse Consulting Firm.

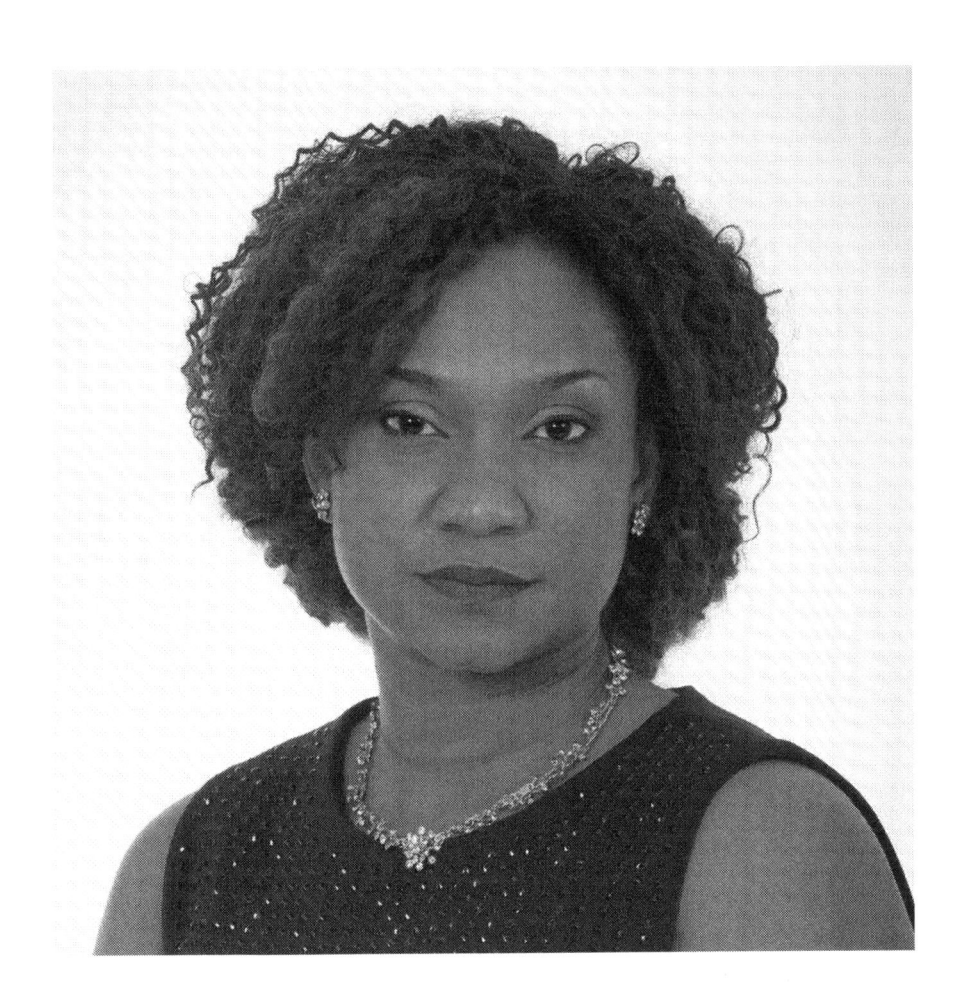

The Blooming Gift

By Malina Spears, LPN

"A society grows great when old women plant trees whose shade they know they shall never sit in." Greek proverb

When I look at the world, I see a giant garden, untamed and overgrown and requiring lots of landscaping and attention. It seems like it's constantly thirsting for more water, more sun and more soil. And so it goes that for me, in a world that's a garden, all the people in it look like unique and beautiful flowers. Of course there are plenty of times when they appear more like weeds. They're hurt or injured or sick, but all that's needed is a little care and some individualized attention for them to transform back into the lovely flowers they are. Unfortunately, in this world, that's not so easy to come by.

Every since I was a little girl, I've been the gardener of people. I spent all of my time caring for others, and I'd never let someone who needed help go without. For me, to see people suffering or in pain would be like walking up to a garden and seeing a wilting daisy with a sagging head. I couldn't and I wouldn't go on walking; I'd make it my duty to give that daisy water until it wasn't wilting anymore.

As I child, I never understood that not everyone saw caring for others as their first priority. It was only as I started to grow up that I saw that there were plenty of people in this world who looked out at a garden and thought nothing of how it got to be so beautiful and full of life. If they saw a plant overgrown with weeds or with dried leaves that needed to be pinched off, they might not stop at all, assuming that things would somehow take care of themselves. Or, perhaps they would simply assume that someone else would be along to care for the plants. Whatever the case, they chose not to interfere, not to stop and help and to just keep walking. I, on the other hand, was born to stop and water the flowers.

Even as I saw and learned more about this type of sentiment, I could never understand it. When I was a little girl, I cared for all of my elderly relatives, as well as my nieces and nephews. When my grandmother got sick, I cared for her, too. At the time, I had twelve living aunts who could've helped in some way, but they were either far away or simply had their own lives to contend with and weren't able to help. As much as I understood this, I couldn't ever imagine opting not to help, regardless of how busy I was. But that, I realized, is something that's unique to the fabric of my being. Not everyone feels this same compulsion to go out of his or her way to help.

When I looked at my grandmother, I saw the woman who was the central figure of our family, but she was also a drinker. I saw that she was suffering and in need of assistance, and my instinct was to do everything I could to help her. It was the same when it came to taking care of my mother, who was in abusive marriages throughout most of my childhood, and I often had to step up and help her, as well. The reflex to help both my grandmother and my mother was second nature to me, and it was this early caretaking that first inspired me to pursue a career in nursing.

I went into home care because my strength was caring for people in tough situations, but what I saw there broke my heart. There are a lot of people working in home care who have the patients' best interests in mind, but there seem to be even more who are there only for the paycheck. Some of the things that I saw during this time distressed me deeply.

I remember walking into one patient's house and there was plenty of food in the cabinets, which was not always the case, but he couldn't eat any of it because he was sharing it all with the rats. I was sickened to see his living conditions, but he couldn't afford anything else. His own children were abusing him mentally, emotionally and financially, and in my position, there was only a limited amount I could do to help. I saw so much mistreatment all the time. It was amazing to me that people could be so cruel to each other. The way the families and other homecare staff would treat patients felt like pouring poison into a beautiful garden. It was so counterintuitive to the field that we were in and the job that we vowed to do.

I tried to do as much as could to help these people, but I felt helpless to do more because it'd be so easy to overstep, and I feared getting fired. I worked hard and did as much as I could while still ensuring not to do anything to jeopardize my job. But it was always a struggle going in day after day and feeling so helpless in the grand scheme of things. I know I'm not the only caring person in the world, but it would sometimes feel like I was, and that burden, that sadness was an excruciating load to bear.

But there were other moments during this time that brought joy to my heart. I met families that took me in as one of their own. One family even invited me on their family vacation, which was very humbling. I also had one resident that begged me to bring my kids to his home on my final visit of the day. I used to visit him and his wife three times daily, and the last visit of the day I'd return to give his wife a bath and put her to bed. The two of them were all alone with all of their children and grandchildren living out of state. It was against company policy, but bringing my children with me on that last visit of the day brought such brightness to this couple's eyes that I couldn't find it in my heart to deny them. As I put his wife to bed, he would make hot chocolates and s'mores for my kids, and they'd sit by the fireplace talking and laughing. He told me this was the best moment of his week. A thing like this may go against policy, but to me, those moments are more healing and joyful than anything written in any manual. And though it was a risk on my part, it was absolutely worth it.

But that's an example of when I was able to do a little something extra to bring joy to my residents. There wasn't always something available for me to do, and that's when I found my job weighed heavily on me. To know what a person needs and be unable to give it to them because of bureaucracy and regulations is what causes the job to start to feel unfulfilling. I felt trapped in a position where I could never do enough. Granted, I know as well as anyone that often it's just those little words of encouragement, or smiles along the way, that mean the most. But even so, it was hard to be satisfied with just those small wins.

I decided I needed to change careers for my own peace of mind, so I got a job in accounting. I figured this was the best move that I could make for myself because it was weighing on me constantly being in this helpless (by my standards) position all the time. I thought an accounting job would pay the bills simply and easily; I could go to work, do my job and then go home without feeling that heavy sense of distress. But my patients kept calling. I always made it a point to give my patients my personal number, just in case something happened. I made it clear that they could all contact me if they wanted. And it turns out, they did. My phone was always ringing.

They'd call me to see how I was doing and would tell me what was going on with them. Then they'd mention the name of someone who passed away or was struggling and would say something like, "No one came." Even though I had tried to remove myself from it all, I found myself getting pulled back in. I was being called back, and it made complete sense to me. After all, my purpose was by no means documenting financial transactions. So, I went back to home care, and I did as much as I could for as long as I could do it.

Eventually, I transitioned into being a traveling nurse, which was a nice change from home care. One of the greatest rewards of being a traveling nurse is the exposure to so many different cultures and walks of life. And for the most part, I was treated well, but there were times when I ran into prejudice. The issues I ran into weren't just about my race, either, but often would have more to do with being a woman. But whatever adversity I ran into, I approached it from a healthy place and just kept doing my job.

Interestingly enough, the lack of care and the neglect that was so prevalent in home care was often just as rampant in the hospitals. As a traveling nurse, you would imagine that because I went wherever I was needed and was always in a different hospital with different patients, that I might be lacking that special touch, that compassionate interaction between nurse and patient. But that was never the case with me, according to my patients. The patients that I treated saw me coming and going. It was evident that my time at a particular hospital was just one stop in a string of many. They'd mention that, and then they'd say, as if they couldn't quite wrap their heads around it, "But it seems like you really care."

And I'd tell them, "That's because I do care."

The reason that they could never really wrap their mind around this was because the nurses that they dealt with that weren't traveling, whose permanent post was in that hospital, and who saw the same patients regularly, were missing that one crucial quality. The majority of nurses interacting with patients have not a shred of compassion to share with their patients. They are there simply doing their job, crossing tasks off of a list and to be honest, are usually pretty overworked and burnt out. But even so, they should be able to manage at least an inkling of true care or compassion. Unfortunately, it was not the case.

And maybe it doesn't have to be. After all, not everyone can be the caretaker or the gardener. But it's the fact that it's not present in every interaction and so often missed that tells me, without a doubt, that this is indeed my true purpose. I was born to see every individual soul as a unique flower in a garden, and I can't walk past a single one without making sure it is cared for and okay.

That's what has led to my ultimate dream, which I am on the brink of achieving. The thing that distresses me the most is when nurses, a profession where the job description literally says caretaker, don't truly care for their patients and don't treat them with the respect that they deserve. I'm now in a position to finally do something about this problem that has been such a big stressor in my life. That's why I'm in the early stages of opening my own assisted living facility in Florida. At my facility, I will no longer have to feel helpless. I won't feel like I'm risking my job every time I try to help, because now I will make the rules. And, of course, my rules will ensure that everyone is cared for at all times and treated with respect. No one will be overlooked or neglected. No one will starve or share their food with rats. The beds won't be viewed as paychecks or invoices, but as people - as beautiful and delicate as flowers. And we'll care for them until we have a beautiful garden of human souls, cared for and healing before us.

I had to delay opening this facility a bit because I am currently struggling with my own sickness. My nature as the caretaker means that I haven't really shared this news with anyone, and my plan has been to just keep moving forward. That's what any true gardener would do, just keep pruning, planting, watering, sowing and weeding. My wellbeing comes from seeing others do well and ensuring others are cared for, so if I can keep doing that, I know that I can get through. My purpose keeps me strong, and every garden needs a gardener.

Biography

A traveling nurse, travel agent and business owner, Malina is a mother to two adult children and five grandchildren. Since the age of 10, she was placed in a caregiver status, while taking care of family and friends. She always knew from an early age that she wanted to be a nurse. As the eldest of five, she had to set an example for all her siblings. She did well in high school, going on to college where she studied business management, while working as a home health aide and nurses aide. With parents that were entrepreneurs, it was instilled in her the importance of having your own business - that way, nobody could dictate your life.

After graduating and starting a homecare business, she felt something was still missing. Malina went on to nursing school at the age of 40. After 10 yrs. of working homecare, nursing homes and assisted living facilities as a nurse, she realized this was where she wanted to be all along. Her plans are continuing to grown in the medical field. Her next step is to open an assisted living facility.

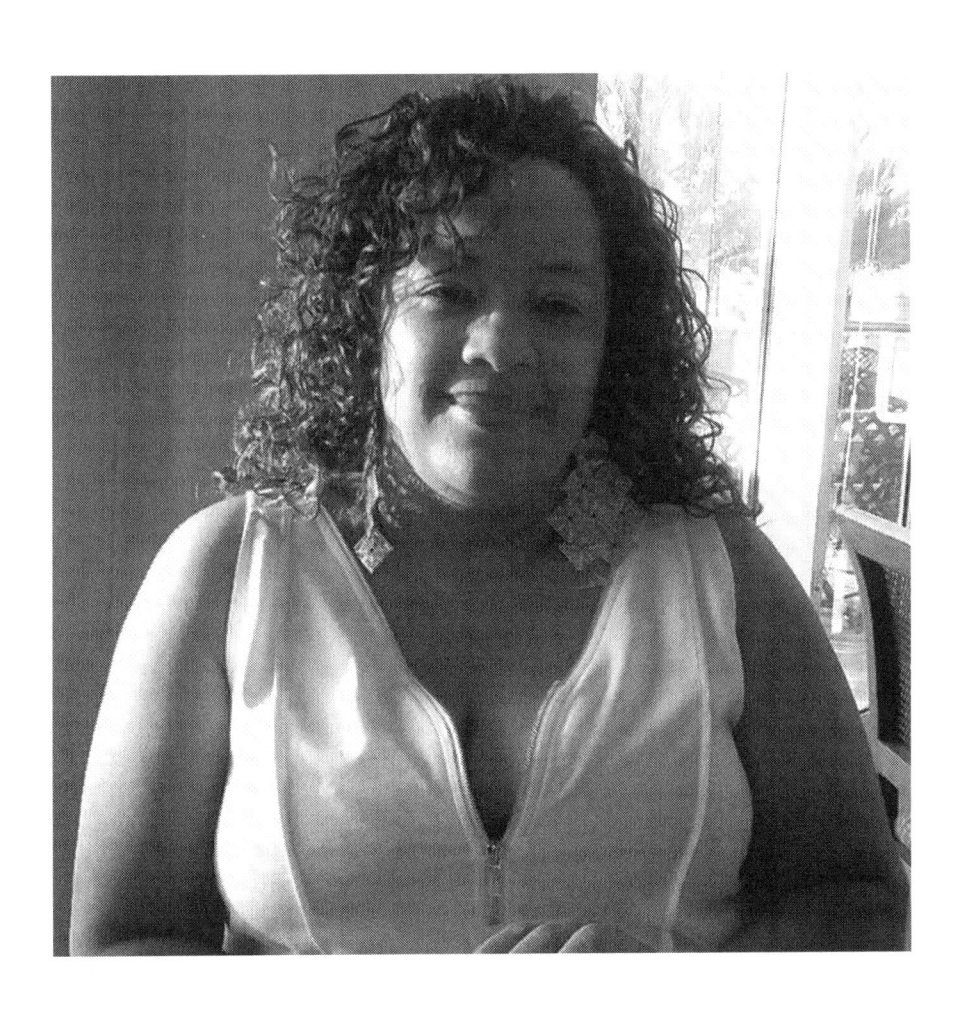

Acknowledgement

Dedicated to all the amazing people who positively impacted my live, prayed and empowered me for greater. Keep inspiring and standing in the gap for others to live in their truth and purpose.

To my momma Janice, thank you for your unwavering support and prayers. You are my wind!

To my sisters Andrea and Felicia, who are no longer with me, you contributed so much to my success. Thank you!

To my husband Darrell, I deeply thank you for your friendship, love, protection and provision. I love you!

Sowing the Seeds of Purpose

By Kecia Hayslett, RN, HTC

"When the purpose of a thing is not known, abuse is inevitable."
~ Myles Munroe

Take that phrase and turn it over in your mind for a moment, and you'll soon see a poignant message embedded there. But it's what that phrase leaves unsaid that is somehow even more magical than what it says. The words we see warn us not to take a thing for granted, but what the phrase only just insinuates is that there is an unimaginable possibility that exists in a thing when you understand that nothing is here by accident, that everything does indeed have a purpose. So, with that in mind, imagine, then, how tragic it is when that inevitable abuse ensues.

Picture, for a moment, a tiny apple seed. From our towering perspective, an apple seed is a miniature coffee been, an insignificant and trivial speck in our much grander existence. So, at a glance, you might decide that the seed is worthless and sweep it away into the trash because it looks like nothing. If you swept that seed away without giving it a second look, you'd have achieved a level of abuse that is astronomical in scope, despite it being such a small action. But, if you had only known in advance their purpose - that those tiny, insignificant seeds would grow into a soaring tree that would provide the fruit that would nourish you and your family - would you have been so quick to sweep those nuisance seeds into the trash?

The thing is, upon seeing seeds for the first time, you wouldn't know their value without a great deal of care and patience. If you refused to put the time in because you were blind to a possible purpose, you would've missed out on something truly amazing. You'd never bite into a crisp, juicy apple on a fall day. It'd be so easy to toss a seed away without proof that it had purpose. But imagine the good that you could do - the joy that you could bring - if you chose to nurture the seed, anyway, in the spirit of assuming there was always some purpose, even if that purpose was invisible to you in the moment.

I started my life as a seed, discarded and neglected, and that feeling of purposelessness lingered for years. Growing up, my biological father used drugs heavily to cope with life after having served in Vietnam. My stepdad was also a Vietnam vet, and he navigated life as a functional alcoholic. Both of these influences rested heavily in my soul and accounted for a lot of pain in my family's daily lives. My mom did her best to protect us, but it was left to me, as the oldest child, to pick up the slack in the areas that were leftover, which mainly included caring for my sister and brothers. I remember how hard my mom tried to show us the possibility of a different life from the one we were living. She would take us to the library as often as possible so that we could travel anywhere in the world we wanted to go. But as hard as she tried to take us away from that problematic home life, and to show us what else was possible in our futures, the trouble was always lurking and remained deeply embedded in my soul.

Because my mother's relationships were laced with such negativity, I also never saw a good, healthy relationship modeled to me. I witnessed clearly my mom's good intentions, but her support of a man who couldn't reciprocate that support stayed with me. It was the only thing I had known. I often found myself picking up the pieces and keeping everyone together and on track when the drinking was heavy and the abuse thick. But I never received any sort of validation from my dad or from my stepdad, so - especially when it came to men - I had no sense of what a healthy, loving relationship looked like. I was young when I got married, mainly

because my religion had taught me that you don't date around; you get married, and once married, you made that marriage work, any way you could. That's all a solid message, but it's a very one-sided view of marriage, because it says nothing of the love that you should have for yourself as well for your partner.

So, I married a boy who paid attention to me and complimented me and made me feel special. But it turned out that I mistook that validation for love. I heard the words for which I had thirsted, and I drank them up. But things changed drastically once our relationship evolved from boyfriend and girlfriend to husband and wife. He had a difficult and abusive childhood, too, but none of that was any excuse for how he treated me. He was physically and verbally abusive; however, I remained passive because I didn't believe in myself enough to stand up to him. Very quickly into the marriage, I had two sons, just one year apart, but even children didn't soften him. He didn't treasure or value any of us, not in a way that was healthy, and I found myself constantly nervous and scared.

Through some of the toughest times in my marriage, my sister was always by my side, supporting me. She'd say, "You don't have to go through that." But though I listened to her and appreciated her concern, the words never sunk in. I never truly believed that I didn't have to go through any of it. After all, I had married him, that had been my choice, and so somehow I must deserve what was coming to me. Plus, whenever things got bad, he'd come back, holding flowers, candy or other gifts, full of apologies…and I'd forget. Or perhaps I just wanted to believe, more than ever, that maybe this time he would change. But he never did.

As a kid, I didn't receive much guidance in terms of what I'd do as a career. The day-to-day of my childhood was so much more focused on survival and simply getting through the next drama, that there was little thought put into the future. But I do remember being encouraged by my aunt. A tiny seed of something was planted when I was a girl watching her work in the court system. As I handled the realities of my own childhood, I watched her life from a distance. I saw that she was powerful and that her job was important. And I remember watching her, thinking, "Wow, if she can do that, what can I do?" I never really had a chance to follow through on this thought until my marriage was already underway. That's when I thought to myself that I'd take my compassionate nature and go back to school for nursing.

I remember one day specifically when I was in class taking an exam. In the middle of that test, an administrator came to the door to interrupt class and told me I had a phone call. At this point, my relationship was already on the rocks. My husband had moved out to an apartment and was not handling the fact that I was pursuing something outside of him very well. The receiver was heavy in my hand as I held it to my ear. It was the police. They were calling about my son, Damian. They said someone had beaten him with a belt and he had welts all over his body. I was terrified. I knew in an instant who was responsible, even though I couldn't believe it. Damian was only five years old at the time, and I felt a rush of anger, hatred and fear all pulsing through me simultaneously. I had to get to him immediately and left my exam behind, unfinished.

I should've left him then, but I didn't. I'm not proud of it, but I simply didn't have the strength or the faith in myself to walk away. Instead, I suppressed all the pain and torment that I was feeling and simply hoped it would go away or change on its own. But it didn't.

The trouble is when you're in an abusive relationship, like the one I was in, the obvious answer to any onlooker is to simply leave, get away from the abuser, start a new life and put that pain behind you. But to the abused, the answer looks a lot different. I thought the answer was that I needed to be better. If I tried harder, if I gave him more, if I made more sacrifices, then he'd finally love me and treat us right, he'd show up for us, he'd change. It always seemed to me that the reason he was acting out was because I was doing something wrong. So even when the problem lay with him, I blamed myself.

A couple of years after the incident with Damian, I was working as a nurse full-time. Money was tight, so I was working long hours to make ends meet. We were living separately at the time, but I still felt it was my job to hold everything together. So, I was paying his bills, his rent and taking care of all of his expenses. I was focusing so much on making sure that he was set that when the first of the month came around, I didn't have enough money leftover to pay my own rent. We were evicted on the spot. That moment was a real wake up call. There had to be a better way, but I was so afraid to ask for a divorce. I was still so mired in his problems, and helping him survive, that I had forgotten about myself and risked my children's well being in the process. I needed to make a change.

We ended up living in the car for a few days until we could find a new apartment. I was trying to figure out a way to leave him, but it turned out I didn't have to. He showed up at my door. Being that close to him, I could feel my heart racing. That fear of him hurting me was still as palpable as ever. He stood there on the step and said, "I need to tell you something. I know you don't want to be with me, so I'm going to ask you for a divorce. I realize that I am not the man for you. You deserve someone who is better than me, who will love you, honor you and not treat you like I have."

Those should have been the most liberating words I had ever heard, but sadly, they weren't. Instead, I felt hurt. He wanted to leave me. He was leaving me. Despite all that he had put me through, I could only feel the rejection and pain of being left. I couldn't hear the part where he was telling me that I deserved better. The only message I received was that he wanted nothing to do with me.

That's how lost I was. I valued myself so little that I was hurt that this abusive man wanted to move on from me. I couldn't see how flawed this view was at the time. I stuffed my feelings down as far as they would go. After the divorce, I stayed away from men altogether. I felt used, abused and mistreated, like there was some sort of gross film on me. Having given so much of myself to a man that could never give anything back left me deeply hurt and scarred. I didn't work through my pain; I just moved it somewhere else.

A couple of years later, my wise, loving and observant sister passed away in a car accident. After that, her husband was stingy and cruel. He wouldn't allow me to participate in her home-going and took my only niece away from me. By this point, my feelings were starting to boil into fine and nasty anger. I was turning into that angry, black woman you see out and about, who is always raving about what's unfair and wrong. I can laugh at that raging stereotype now, but then I was so full of anger and blame that I was unrecognizable. I was in so much pain that I'd stay awake all night, eating. There were nights I'd eat a whole chocolate cake or an entire bag of cookies, all by myself. I tried to eat away the pain, to fill myself with something other than the torment I was feeling, but nothing worked.

I woke up one morning, alone in my bed, and it hit me like a truck – the loneliness was more palpable than ever. I realized I had absolutely no one to call; no one with whom to have a coffee with; no one to talk to. There was not a single person I could reach out to if I needed a shoulder to cry on or even just a ride to the store. That feeling was absolutely debilitating and flat-out scary. I sat there for a bit, frozen. Then, a voice came from somewhere inside of me. It sounded like my sister's, and it said, "You can change this."

At that point, I fell to the floor, in the fetal position, and just cried. I cried hard for an hour or more. Every feeling, every emotion, every unheard plea poured out of me. Something in me broke that day, and in that breakdown, a new attitude swept over me. As I lay there weeping, I decided to forgive myself and to forgive others. I'd finally shed the blame that I had insisted on carrying around for so long. I wrote a pile of letters to the people closest to me who had let me down, and in the letters, I forgave them all. As soon as I got everything out of my system, I balled up the letters, threw them into the fireplace and watched them burn. The house reeked of ash and smoke, but those heavy feelings were lifted away. It was like thirty pounds had been lifted off my shoulders. My new motto was to deal and feel. Never again was I going to ignore my feelings and stuff them down.

Even with that big realization and change of attitude, I still needed a push when it came to my career. I was working on the nurse floor one day when an unforgettable incident occurred. Prior to the incident, I had been having these dreams where I'd encounter this person, who was the physical representation of my dreams, sitting in a chair in the corner of my basement, with duct tape on her mouth. In the dream, the person was shouting through the duct tape, "When will you untape me?" The dream ended with me running upstairs. I didn't think too much about it until this patient on my floor started having a reaction. I remember locking eyes with her, and it was as if we were communicating without saying a word. She started slipping away and began to code. I ran over and knelt alongside her and whispered the simplest thing in her ear. I said, "You will live and not die." Then her eyes closed and she was rushed off to ICU.

About one week later, that same woman found me. "You don't know, but you saved my life," she said. She went on to say that she couldn't talk during that moment, but she could hear, and it was my kind words that stayed with her and pulled her through. This all brought me back to the dream that I had the previous week. I thought to myself that if I could do that for her, I surely could do that me, and for my own dream of starting my business. The entire incident directly inspired me to get out of my own way and start my homecare business. And since then, I've started other consulting and training businesses, as well. I know that I have an important message to share, and it's my duty and purpose to share it.

Forgiving myself was a critical step on the way to fulfilling my purpose. Once I was able to release all those feelings of worthlessness and shame, I suddenly realized what value I could bring to the world. I realized that for my entire life, I was waiting for permission: permission to succeed, permission to feel loved, permission to be me. When I received validation, I'd place too much stock in it and give that person too much power over me, and it would usually always backfire. What I've since learned is that validation has to start with me. The only person who needs to believe in me is me, and by loving myself first, I'm able to give more to others. I'm able to live my purpose, which is to help alleviate suffering in others.

I've also learned that fostering a spirit of non-forgiveness and blame only detracts from my true path. When you focus on everything that is wrong in the world, that's all that you'll see. The power lies in all of us to create our own joy. We choose how we see the world and how we view others. We create our own reality with the language that we use and the things we choose to focus on, and if you can find a way to cultivate joy in your everyday life, you'll find that happiness is the byproduct of that process.

My mission now is to make sure that others understand that they are here for some purpose. At first, it doesn't matter if you know what that purpose is - just know that it does exist. And more importantly, following your purpose is not a selfish endeavor that requires validation from others before you can get started. Following your purpose is the most selfless act you can do, because when you're following it, you most certainly are benefiting and edifying others along the way. We are all born with the tiny seeds of our purpose inside of us. They were planted there long before our birth, and it is up to us to water those seeds, let them grow, protect them from harm and become who we are meant to be.

Biography

Kecia Hayslett, a family girl with humble beginnings, is a graduate of The Nursing program at The College of Saint Catherine.

Chemotherapy, Medical-Surgical, Acute Care, Case Management and Home Health Care are the many areas of Nursing she has worked.

Today, Kecia has found success as a nurse entrepreneur; a loving family and a life well lived. After years of studies and countless hours on her feet as a nurse, Kecia embarked upon her entrepreneurial journey with Excellence Health Career Center, a stationary and mobile health career training center created to educate, equip and empower the aspiring health care worker for entry level jobs in the healthcare field.

Now the founder of S.N.A.P. Soulful Nurses Activating Purpose, Kecia works tirelessly to promote work-life synergy with the purpose of promoting events, online programs and workshops to help nurses learn to maximize their gifts and talents.

Kecia Hayslett is a wife, mother, nona (grandma), speaker and author.

Connect and learn more at

Website: www.KeciaHayslett.com

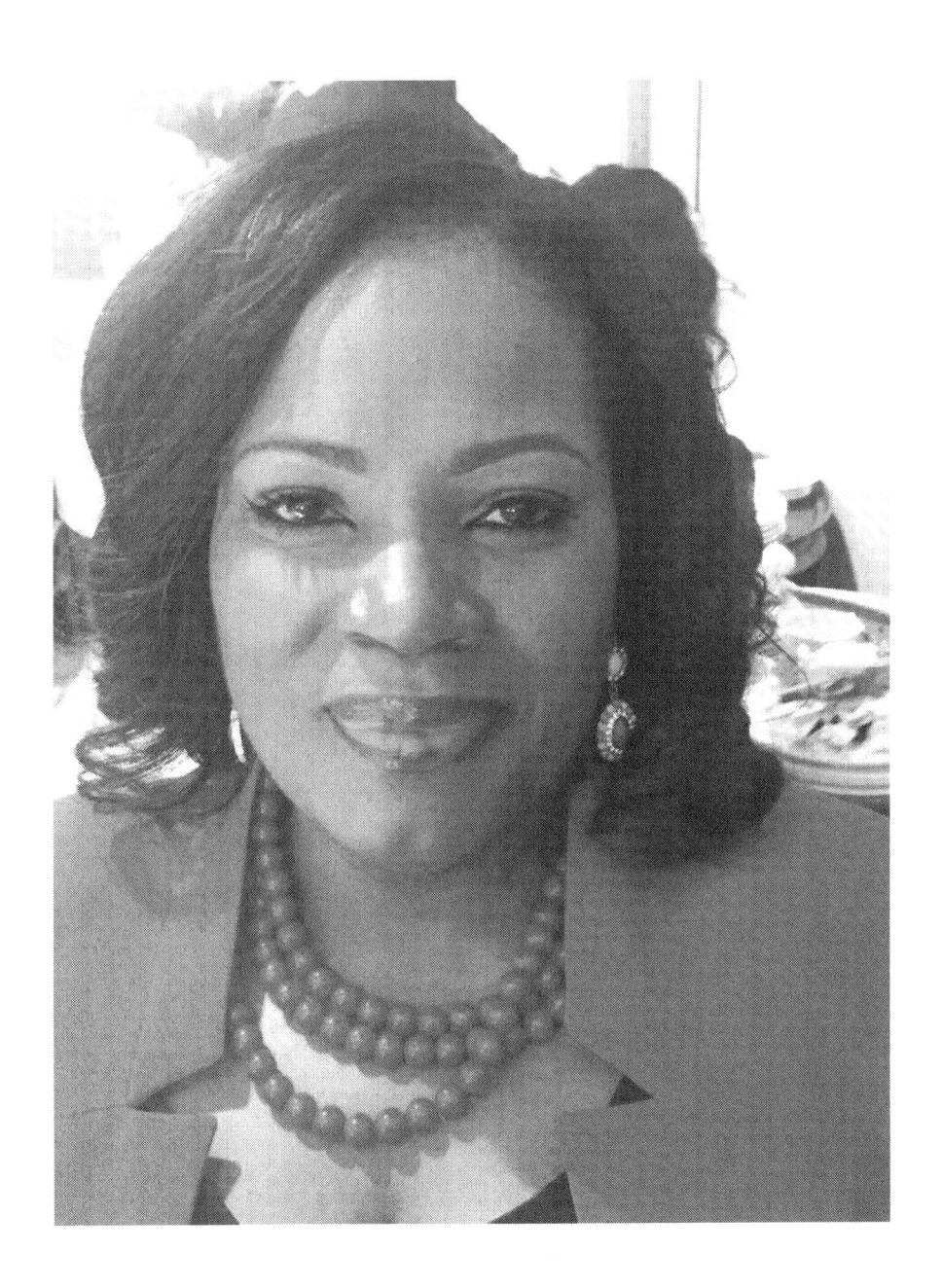

Acknowledgements

I would like to dedicate this book to my beautiful children: Tinia, Landen, Liyanna, Re'Asia, La'Vern IV. You all have been my strength and motivation throughout this entire process. The legacy I seek to build is for ALL for you.

To my loving husband La'Vern Payne III. You are truly a blessing to me, thank you for believing in me and for your constant support. I love you.

To my beautiful mother Ernestine, words can't express how much I appreciate you for ALWAYS being in my corner and pushing me towards my purpose. Your unconditional love and encouragement is the reason I never gave up.

I give thanks to GOD for answering my prayers and using me to help and motivate others.

~Tina

Push Past Your Fear and Find Your Purpose: A Woman's Anthology to Power

By Tina Marie Payne, MSN, RN

Fear is deceptive. It leaks into your subconscious and will take up permanent residence there if you let it. It will seep into every thought, every effort and every endeavor. It will weaken what it touches until those thoughts are no more than distant memories pinned to a vision board in the corner of your room somewhere. Many women allow fear to paralyze them and stop them from fulfilling their true desires. Fear is the reason distractions start to look so appealing to us. Even when we know in our gut what path we want to follow, sometimes those cracks in the façade, those fears about our inadequacy or our inability to achieve start to creep in. These fears nudge us off our path and away from our God-given purpose. We welcome the shiny distractions, and sometimes that's enough to completely change our direction.

But I am here to tell you that this doesn't have to be the case. The trick to combating fear lies in finding our true purpose, and living in accordance with the path that resonates. Above all else, we need to keep that purpose safe. We need to treasure it with all of our strength and call it back when it strays. When we are following our true purpose, we don't have to be scared. Sometimes, we just need a little help remembering. I know this only because I lived through it. At three different points in my life, I was beaten down and rocked by fear. Three times I found myself in the dark, with nothing to guide me out but my own will. And all three times, I faced my pain and persisted. But it was never easy. And I could only really see the value of getting through those times from the other side. That's why my story is so important. I want to share with others how crucial it is to persist, to move through the distractions, to shake the fear and to do what you were meant to do, no matter how difficult the first step.

"Everything you want is on the other side of fear." – Jack Canfield

As a teenager in high school, I knew exactly what I wanted to do with my life. I wanted to be a doctor, ever since I can remember, so I worked hard in school with that goal in mind. I graduated in the top ten percent of my high school and was accepted to all three of the Ohio universities to which I applied. I settled on one that was about an hour away from my hometown and signed up for courses that would put me on the track for pre-med. So, that first year, I majored in biology and was making great progress.

My grades were good, I had lots of great friends and I was truly enjoying the freedom of living on my own. But things can change in an instant. At the end of my first year of college, I found out I was pregnant. The news felt like squealing brakes on a highway. One minute I was cruising down the freeway; the next I was tripped up on the side of the road. I looked out my window at all my peers walking to their classes, and suddenly I was no longer one of those happy-go-lucky students. I had been in college nearly nine months, and in another nine months, I'd have a newborn baby.

I was scared because in that moment, I knew my life would change forever. Having a baby is scary when you're prepared for it, and here I was, still a kid myself, with a list of big dreams in front me that were now not viable. I was scared because I didn't know how

I was going to support a child and continue my education. And deep down, I was even more fearful that I was about to become another statistic, not only letting myself down, but everyone around me. It didn't seem fair. I had worked so hard up until this point, and in an instant, my entire course was altered. I was not invincible. I was not safe from the ups and downs of life just because I had these big plans for the future.

The easy choice was sitting right in front of me. I could move back home in an instant. My parents were insisting on it, and I knew that they had the best intentions; but I also knew that if I moved home, I'd be doing myself a disservice. I'm sure things would have been fine, but that's all they would've been – just fine. I knew, deep down, that I couldn't go home – not if I wanted to make something of myself. The comfort and safety of home would have been like putting sand on that fire to succeed, burning within me. I wouldn't need to push myself at home; I could transfer to a community college. But would I really continue on my desired path? To go home at that point in my life would've meant giving up on me and doing what was best for my child in that moment. But would that really be what was best for my child in the long run? Something inside of me didn't think so. I knew that I needed to make my original intention work somehow. There had to be another way that I could stay on track, stay in school and have my baby.

It was clear to me at this point that it wasn't realistic to think that I could continue on a pre-med path. That'd be way too intense and rigorous now that I had two of us to worry about, but that didn't mean I had to abandon the field altogether. That's when I decided on nursing. Going into the nursing profession made complete sense to me. It was not far off from being a doctor and would still allow me the opportunity to work in a compassionate capacity and serve as a patient advocate, two things that I knew were important to me. Plus, I knew it offered a stable income, the potential for long-term financial growth and that in my current state, the schooling required would be more manageable to balance with being a single mother than my original pre-med plans.

So, that's what I chose - nursing. I was lucky in a lot of ways. My college had family housing available, so although I was put on the waiting list initially, I didn't have to look for alternative housing arrangements and was in a two-bedroom unit by the time my daughter arrived. Plus my friends and family were close enough in proximity that they could help me with my daughter when needed. During the first three months, I reduced my schedule to part-time as I acclimated to being a new mother. I kept my course load manageable with two classes that met only once a week.

That first summer, while I picked up a job as a nurse's aid working the night shift, I enrolled my daughter in a daycare program that was open twenty-four hours a day. It made me feel a little bit better that she was mostly asleep during the hours I was gone, and I wasn't missing that much awake time with her, even though the night shift is never easy. Then, when school started, I enrolled her in daycare during my class hours. But even so, sometimes I had no choice but to bring her to class with me. I was always worried that she'd be disruptive, but there was nothing I could do. I still remember the cold, judgmental stares I got from my classmates. I know what I looked like to them, and it was tough to hold my head up high at times. What they didn't know was how terribly thin the difference between us was and how it could've been any one of them in my shoes instead. It just happened to be me.

Nothing about going through nursing school with a baby was simple, and I had to make many sacrifices that I wouldn't have had to make otherwise. The daycare closed at 6pm some nights, but my classes didn't end until 7pm, meaning I'd have to miss an entire hour of those classes to get there in time. Because of all the time I was missing, I ended up having to retake some of those classes, and I utilized my parents' help whenever I could for the times when I needed longer studying sessions.

Even with all the effort I was putting in, it still wasn't quite enough. One spring morning, I read the cold, typed words of a letter that said I hadn't passed and was being kicked out of the nursing program. My heart sank. Here I was, working as hard as I could, but felt like I was getting nowhere. I really wanted to give up at that point. I felt overwhelmed and questioned whether or not I should even stay in school. After crying and feeling sorry for myself for a few days, I asked God to show me the way. I remembered that I was capable; that I deserved to be there, and giving up was not the answer. So, I went into action mode. I worked hard to appeal the nursing board's decision, and I had everyone who could write letters on my behalf. I remember my mom telling me, "Tina Marie, God has the final say, no matter what the appeal board decides. God can always work in your favor."

Through the grace of God, six months later, I was readmitted on a probationary basis, and I knew I could not blow this second chance. That entire process instigated a lot of fear in me. I hated that my life was in the hands of these decision makers who had no idea what life was like in my shoes. I was doing the best that I could, but still I was completely at their mercy. In 2004, I walked proudly across that graduation stage, my three-year-old daughter right there with me.

"The question isn't who is going to let me; it's who is going to stop me."
— Ayn Rand

When I look back on those times, I'm not quite sure how I made it through, how I balanced raising a baby with going to school and working to support her. I think that I did it all because I knew I had no other choice, and that the sacrifices in the present would mean a better future for both of us. But even now, it really hits me how close I was to giving up. At any time, I might've just reached my breaking point and given up on my dream. If I had made one different decision, or let myself believe that the sacrifices I was making at the time just weren't worth it, I might be in a totally different place today. I didn't allow fear of failure to overtake me. Sure, it would've been easier for me if I had my first daughter later in life, but in retrospect, I wouldn't change a thing. Our struggle early on helped make us who we are today and paved the way for dealing with the hardships yet to come.

After I graduated from nursing school, my daughter and I relocated two hours away from my hometown, and I ended up getting married. During that marriage, I had two more children, but it wasn't until after my third child that I entered a really dark time in my life. I remember clear as day lying in my bed, staring up at the ceiling fan in my bedroom. But I wasn't just looking at it and watching the propellers spin round and round. I was analyzing what it was made of. I studied the propellers and imagined their weight, thought about their color, and how they were built; then I wondered if they could hold me. I saw the image of my own body and imagined what it might look like hanging from those propellers. I was literally thinking about ways to hang myself. My husband was right downstairs with the children and here I was, feeling glued to the bed, trapped, like a magnet had me and wouldn't let go. The physical and mental anguish I was feeling at that time of my life had me believing that the world, my family and my children would be better off without me. I just wanted the pain to go away. I lay there for hours, as if I was a part of the bed. I cried out to God to help me and fell asleep, repeating it over and over.

That wasn't my first suicidal thought, either. Just a few weeks before, I had pulled into my garage, closed the door and just sat there for a few minutes, wondering…hoping…that the room would fill with a toxic gas that would just silence this overwhelming apathy I was feeling. How easy it would be to just pass out and disappear. But then my phone rang and vibrated in my lap, which somehow snapped me back into reality. What was I doing? What was I thinking? Any honest look at my life would suggest that I had so much to live for – three children, a husband, a new house, a good job. But depression seeps into your mind and body and doesn't let go. There's no reasoning with that level of depression. And what's scariest about it is that you're so used to relying on yourself and changing your perspective when things are tough, that the inability to do that leaves you feeling trapped, like you have no way out. With depression, you've got nothing to give, nothing seems worth the effort, and you're so deep into that hopeless state that it's impossible to imagine anything different.

The depression really just snuck up on me, and at first, I didn't even understand that it was depression. I knew I had physical pain and mental anguish that just wouldn't let go, but the diagnosis came later. I wondered - how could I, as a nurse, not recognize my own symptoms? I didn't want to tell anyone what was going on in my mind. I was fearful of judgment, and I was ashamed. But because I was a nurse, I knew I couldn't tell my patients to get help and then not follow my own advice. So I did; I got professional help.

Telling my mom made it even more real, but she came through and supported me beyond words. She knew that I needed a change of environment, so she arrived at my doorstep to take me away from my house and responsibilities and simply took care of me for a few weeks

At the time, I was enrolled in a Master's program and working as a hospice nurse, which were both not helping my current state of mind. I removed myself from both of those environments. It was so important to remove all of the stressors from my life so that I didn't have anything to worry about except getting myself healthy and back into a positive state of mind. Some of the most important things during that time became my rituals, like journaling, going on walks, writing prayers, reading my bible and repeating self-affirmations. Connecting with my family members and closest friends was also very powerful. Living life two hours away from my foundation had left me feeling isolated and alone. My husband was not very supportive, and maybe he didn't know how to be. Either way, I felt like I alone had the burden of caring for the kids. The move to focus on me for this period of time was instrumental in helping me get back on my feet.

When I look back at this depression, I see that the fear had caught up with me. I was overwhelmed and felt like I was alone in my life.

Just like when I was pregnant with my oldest daughter, I knew that changing my environment would make or break me. The first time, going home would have derailed my dreams. But now, going home was essential, at least for a little while. I needed to change the scene and shift the focus to my own self-care, rather than giving all my energy to others.

Part of the reason why that depression took such a hold of me was because of my marriage. Maybe I idealized it and told myself that everything was okay, but it was far from perfect. I should've heeded the warning signs early on. I remember a time in the beginning when, over some trivial disagreement, he threw his wedding ring at me. But I always assumed things would change; that he would get better with time. But once we had kids, it became even harder to leave and nothing changed. He was verbally and mentally abusive and never came through as the supportive partner and co-parent for which I had hoped.

I was fearful about what I would say to the children, and fearful that others would judge me. The fears had me paralyzed and unwilling to make a move. About eight years into the marriage, I felt lost and worn. I had withstood a lot of disrespect and given so much of myself to this man, with nothing coming back in return, that I needed some sort of change. I repeatedly asked him for some space and time to think about our future. I didn't do it in a hurtful way. It was simply a request that I needed to be granted for me as a person, but he didn't like that and refused to give me what I asked for. He wouldn't stand for even one day apart. After months of me asking, he finally came upstairs one morning before work and said, "Okay, I'll leave. I'll give you your time."

Not five minutes later, I heard crashing sounds on the first floor. I went running downstairs to see family picture frames strewn across the floor, furniture upturned and all of my degrees crashed and broken in a pile. My children were standing there, crying and holding on tightly to their book bags. His anger was horrifying, and I took the kids back upstairs with me and locked them safely in their rooms. I called 911, my mom and my boss to say I wouldn't be coming in that day.

When the police arrived, there was very little that they could do. They couldn't tell either one of us to leave, and he wasn't budging, only threatening. He said to me in a stern voice, "You need to get out of my house." So, while the police stood there, I gathered up the kids, told them to put everything they could fit into trash bags, and we left. As we exited through the garage, he called out after us, "The locks will be changed; don't think you're coming back," and I knew he didn't have to bother with the locks. There was no chance we were going anywhere near him again.

But just like my other decisions, leaving him was the best option; it just wasn't the easiest. We had nowhere to go initially, but my mom helped me find a small apartment not too far from the kids' school. We slept on the floor for a few weeks until I could get furniture. We stayed there for six months while I filed for divorce. After the courts granted me the rights, we moved back to my hometown, Cincinnati, and stayed with my mother for a period of time. As hard and messy as it got, my children were my driving factor. I knew I had to do whatever I could to make things okay for them. It was challenging, because I grew up believing that you do whatever you can to make your marriage work. Part of me was disappointed that I was unable to succeed at that, but in the end, I was glad - I needed to show my kids that the better option was being the stronger woman and leaving.

"You gain strength, courage and confidence by every experience in which you really stop to look fear in the face. You must do the thing which you think you cannot do." — Eleanor Roosevelt

My cousin, a marriage counselor, gave me some great advice that has stuck with me: "It's okay to start your life over; you can give yourself that permission." That was so important for me to hear. Sometimes, you feel like you work so hard to get your life going in the right direction that it seems like you're doing irreparable damage to everything you've worked for when you change course, when you get a divorce, when you make a big move or make a life-altering decision. But the truth is, you can start your life over at any time.

"Fear defeats more people than any other one thing in the world."
— Ralph Waldo Emerson

Whoever is reading this, if you get nothing else from my story, please get this: never let fear stop you from following your purpose in life. You're not locked into one direction just because you set out that way. We're free to change, to adapt, to reorganize our lives based on what's happening in the present. There's no need to stay in yesterday especially if it doesn't suit you today.

Letting that sink in really helped me after my divorce. I started a business during the final year of my marriage, but had to stop as I went through this transition. Once I came back home, I was ready to re-launch it with a totally new mission and a newfound strength.

I no longer had to worry about this man putting me down and taking energy away from my pursuits.

Since that time, I've started multiple successful businesses, entered into a new, healthy relationship in which I'm supported and cared for, and we now have five children, total. Life right now is everything I imagined it to be. I run my own business, I coach others in similar situations, I homeschool three of my children and I'm grateful for everything that I have. But the truth is that even if something difficult were to come along again, I've got the resources now to handle anything that comes my way.

Every trial that has come before has prepared me for where I am now. I don't look back on the hard times in my life and feel sad about them. Rather, I am grateful for them because they've all helped make me into the strong and resilient woman I am today. **I don't allow fear to be a factor.** The fear I felt in my marriage, the fear I felt during my depression that afternoon so long ago and the fear that I had when I found out I was pregnant that very first time - that fear is simply a nemesis that I've fought and beaten. And I know if I did it once, twice, three times, that it no longer wields any power over me. I don't allow it to sway me. Fear is only as powerful as YOU allow it to be, and distractions can only take you as far away from your dreams as you let them. I no longer look at tough times as something to be feared. I embrace the difficult because I know I'm strong enough to handle anything that comes my way…and I continue on, living my purpose.

Biography

Tina M. Payne is a graduate of the University of Phoenix, with a Masters in Nursing Education. She successfully obtained her Bachelors of Science Degree in Nursing at Wright State University. Tina has worked as a registered nurse for 14 years in a variety of areas including, hospice, progressive care, emergency room, telemetry and also as a Nursing instructor. To maintain her nursing skills Tina still maintains a nursing position at a local hospital.

Since 2013, Tina M. Payne has also found success away from the bedside as the CEO of two businesses: Grace Health Career Center, a health career-training center, and Grace Health Scrubs, a mobile and online uniform store. Combining her own entrepreneurial background with the desire to motivate and empower other women, she created an online group, *Goals of a CEO Mom*. The overwhelming response from members of the group quickly expanded to Tina offering coaching services to other nurses who desire to create their dream business so they can live a fulfilled life beyond the bedside.

Tina has demonstrated leadership in her community, she currently serves on the on the board of her local chapter of *Black Nurses Rock Cincinnati*, as the Marketing, Media, and Membership Director. Black Nurses Rock is national non-profit organization that aims to inspire, empower and educate those in underserved communities.

Tina, the nurse, author, speaker and entrepreneur, attributes a lot of her personal motivation and drive to her loving husband and five beautiful children. Part of Tina's motivation to work from home was so that she could homeschool her children. Tina enjoys spending time with her family and traveling to new places, she especially loves the beach and the mountains.

Connect with Tina for that extra push towards your purpose, business coaching, or speaking engagements:

Website: www.tinampayne.com

Email: Tina@goalsofaceomom.com

Facebook: www.facebook.com/goalsofaceomom

LinkedIn: www.linkedin.com/in/tinampayne/

Instagram: www.instagram.com/goalsofaceomom

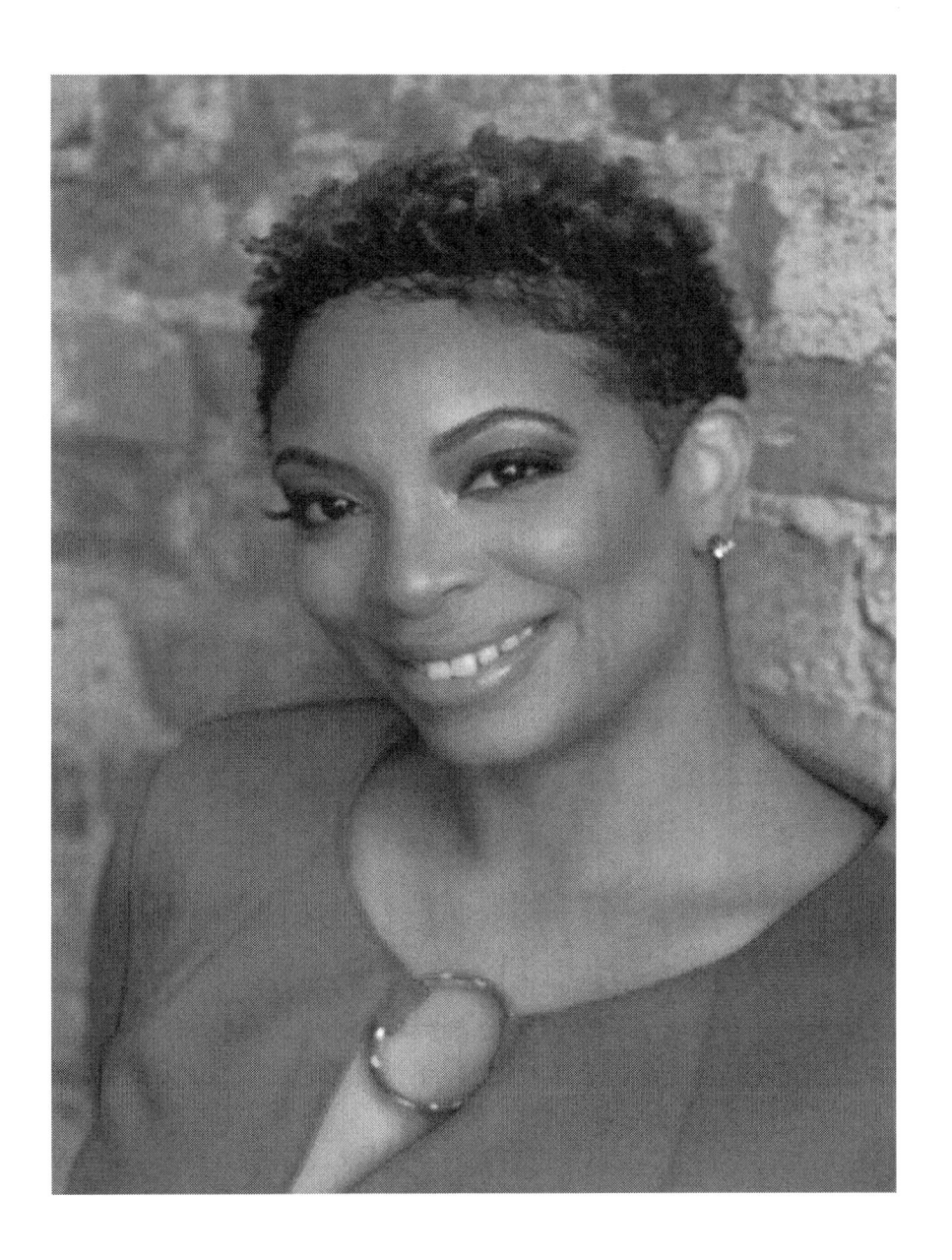

Acknowledgements

Dedicated to the black and brown women in white, my parents, John and Earlene Smiley, my clan and siblings who have always been by my side. Thank you for your unconditional love, which I accept and humbly give back. My nursing instructors, who taught me the power of education, to my mentors, Retta Zeigler, who supported me in the quest to teach, Stella Nsong, who added fuel to my fire so that all the colors burned bright, and to Michelle Rhodes, who steered me along a path to repurpose my existing knowledge.

"I don't want nobody to give me nothing, to open the door, I will get it myself."

James Brown, Godfather of Soul

BEGINNINGS:

An Anthology for Women Acknowledging their gifts

By Willa Smiley, MSN, MEd., RN, CCM, LNC

I've always been drawn to precious stones. Diamonds, emeralds, rubies and others sparkling from beneath jewelry counters. As they are demystified in the pages of science textbooks, they have always caught my attention and sparked my imagination. The reason goes far beyond the stones' physical beauty or worth. In looking at these stones and rolling them around between my fingers, I feel a deeper connection, I can relate to their rich history and creation. At a glance, they almost seem to good to be true. Basically, their entire existence relies solely upon a certain cluster of ingredients going through a particular set of conditions. Ultimately, it's the fact that these minerals underwent exceptionally stressful conditions in order to become gems rather than the "old dirt" they are made of. It's such a consoling thought to think that in order for these beautiful specimens to exist, they need make it through a tumultuous period of high pressure and intense heat. It's only after they go through these stressors and come out the other end, that they emerge, rare and beautiful, and uncharacteristically strong despite this delicate beauty. It seems against all odds, and perhaps that's why I feel such kinship and connection to these miraculous creations – because I know all too well what it's like to move through tumultuous times and emerge as rare and precious as a gem.

I was born in a small gladiolus farming town called Little Harlem, situated on the Gulf of Mexico. The season was fall, but it was nothing like the picturesque New England falls you'd recognize from magazines where the leaves change to beautiful ambers and reds, and the air is just brisk enough to provide a refreshing boost to the spirit after a sweltering summer. Fall here wasn't a quick relief. It was a gentle lessening, a dull subsiding. The days were getting shorter, but they were still hot, almost like the season itself acknowledged the shorter presence of the sun, but refused to relent as a matter of principal. It didn't matter that the world wanted it to be less intense, it would still burn bright until it was ready to cool down on its own.

I entered the world with a similar sense of defiance and an almost predestined knowledge of my own schedule. My aunt was pregnant with her fourth child at the same time that my mom was pregnant with me. As luck would have it, my dad took my aunt the midwife in town to give birth, but just as his car edged around the bend, the labor pains struck. My mom called another nearby aunt to come and help, but by the time she arrived, her and I were already in the shower in the midst of the birthing process. Right from the start, I had proven that I didn't wait for external conditions to be right. I was on my timeline. When I was ready to do something, it was time. This was a gift I had from day one.

I am a progression of humble beginnings. Early on, my parents, siblings and I lived in three-room apartment in Fort Myers. My parents slept in the living room, and my siblings and I shared a foldout and a double bed in the bedroom. There was a modest kitchen with a sink and small, enclosed room with a toilet, but not much beyond that.

Being poor as a child was not difficult in the way it's difficult for an adult. Being poor was all we knew, so we adapted just fine. The thing that makes an impression though is the discovery that you're different from other people, and that there's this giant chasm between everything you know and everyone else. The realization comes slowly too, in dribs and drabs. It's little things, like never reading a story with a character who resembles you, realizing you're the only one who is seeing milk in a carton for the first time, and the awareness that I on most days wore a red dress to school while others seemed to have more variety in their wardrobes.

Eventually, we moved out of Fort Myers and back to Harlem, but the house we moved to was just a shell of a home, nothing more. The rooms only had half of their walls, and the toilet wasn't installed. We had to use a bucket and every morning or night, my big brother would empty it in the bushes. Early after this move, I remember going to the store with my Dad. Out of the corner of my eye, I saw a woman with her child, and I remember being struck at the difference. Their skin and hair was an entirely different color. This was the first time I had seen a white person, and I stopped and turned all the way around to get a better look. My Dad pulled on my hand to keep up, but still I couldn't help but think, "how strange." I didn't say a word, just thought about it and recognizing the sensation of being different, that's what I was wasn't the only thing to be.

During our time in Harlem, they were breaking ground on new elementary school, Heights Elementary. Once completed, it would serve the entire community. There'd be a classroom for each grade, and it was for all the kids I knew around the neighborhood. By the time I was in fifth grade, I was really looking forward to finally being the one of the leaders as well as being in the 6th grader. This school was where I belonged, and it felt like home to me. But I never got the chance of being a leader in the 6th grade at Heights Elementary. This was the start of a time of what I call "forced integration." It was the end of the latter part of the 60s, and Heights Elementary School was a casualty of this new social movement. The change was abrupt. One day we were students at Heights, and the next day, there were locks and chains around the school. It was as if it was some sort of dangerous or restricted area. Up until that point, parents used to be able to choose what school they wanted to send their kids to, but this year- things would be different. All in the spirit of this "integration." My fate would be determined based on what side of the street we lived on. Unfortunately for me, I was the only black girl who lived on a side of the street that determined my new school to be Fort Myers Beach Elementary.

Much like it sounds, Fort Myers Beach Elementary School was a white school catering to the white kids who lived on Fort Myers Beach. I had heard lots of stories about going to school with white kids. "They will bet you up," "They will put your head in the toilet," and other horrifying warnings. As the bus drove up, and we stepped onto the pavement outside the school, the penetrating stares were palpable. The white kids were looking at us, the newcomers, and all we could do was stare back. From the bus, we were directed to the cafeteria where we would then find out where are classrooms were. When my name was called, a little girl got up and said she'd take me to my classroom. Of the three of us that were from my side of the street, I was the only black girl, and I turned out to be the only black girl in the sixth grade. I felt my dreams of being a leader, being in charge, and being looked up to at my old school melt away.

When I got to my classroom, my teacher, Mrs. Head, put her arms around me and welcomed me to her class. She pointed me toward a seat in the middle row toward the back of the room. I felt all of the stares of all the kids boring holes into my back as clutched tightly onto my notebook and moved toward my seat. During recess, I watched as all the blonde-haired, blue-eyed kids laughed and joked with each other. They talked about their weekends playing on the beach and riding on their parents' boats. They weren't saying anything negative or positive outright mean to me. However, I felt impossibly different from these kids and terribly alone. I also couldn't understand why the differences existed. Had I done something to deserve it? My weekends consisted of working on the gladiolus flower farm. I'd lug flowers back and forth (because I was still to young to do the cutting) in order to give the adults some time off. I would wonder, was this new my reality … me a being a laborer on a flower farm while my new colleagues enjoyed themselves on beaches and in boats and jet-stetted to different countries for entire semesters?

No one ever made real on those threats of putting my head in the toilet or beating me up, but still the toll of being so different from peers took a huge toll on me. At a time of life when kids need acceptance and a shared experience more than anything else, it was difficult to reconcile. Because the differences between me and my peers was so striking, it made me feel as if something about me was inferior. What was supposed to be a wonderful integration of blacks and whites served only to highlight everything that was different about me. It left me feeling ashamed and distant. I purposefully made the decision to NOT integrate. It felt like it would be an abandonment of my culture to even try, not that I'd even have been successful if I did make an attempt. I'm sure the optics of the effort looked great when you saw it from a distance. How great it is that they were attempting to unite black and white kids together in schools after so much time being separated, but it was still so early. There might've been a lot to gain on a global level, but at the microcosmic level of one black girl forced to go to school with a classroom of white kids, the devastation was catastrophic.

This was just one awkward era of many awkward times in my life, but it shaped and molded me in ways that can't be undone. I moved through those years in a daze, and I stayed introspective, asking myself questions like, "is this my new world?" and "can I survive it?"

As the years went on, integration got a little easier because more black people started to show up. We were by no means common in our school, but we at least had the beginnings of a community, and we weren't entirely alone in our experiences. Things were fun, uneventful, and there were enough of us that I had friends again. I was able to relax my defenses and explore a little.

When you go through such a visceral experience of being alone, you tend fall harder into the outstretched arms of friends when you find them. This could be how I ended up pregnant for the second time by the time I was 16 years old. I remember walking home from school, and feeling suddenly dizzy and tired. I turned onto my street, and palpable sensation came over me. I wondered, "who am I and what am I here for… am I really living or am I just existing?" As I got closer to my parents' house, I opted not to go inside. I went around the back steps instead and sat down. I looked up into the bushes and stared at how they faded off into the horizon. This wasn't me. I had never been the kind of person who let life direct me and relinquished having an active role. Sure I was stuck at the moment, in this sort of pre-ordained existence where there didn't seem to be a lot of options or support. But I was gifted. I was smart. And I had a passion, though very buried, to accomplish things.

I thought harder, and I thought about my skin color. And though maybe based on my circumstances and the times (it was still only the 70s by now,) I should've been ashamed, I wasn't. I was black, and I was proud of it. My parents, my grandparents, my clan of siblings, we were all smart, loving and hard-working people, and there was no shame in that. Even this pregnancy and being a woman felt like the world was trying to put another burden onto me, but I didn't feel ashamed of that either. I didn't feel that being a woman made me weaker. My current child was already the source of so much strength and love, and this next one on the way would only add to that.

It wasn't in my interest to continue going to school. At the time, it felt like that the external environment was only pushing me farther away from myself. What I needed was a least a few months, to simply think, to figure out who I was and where I needed to go so I could follow my own true purpose and life path.

In retrospect, I think that this hiatus was me "crystallizing" much like the dirt and minerals need time to turn into precious gems. I had made it through some pressures, some boiling point, and some tremulous situations, and now I just needed to crystallize. I took this time to really reflect on my life and the situations that lead me to where I was. I thought back to first grade. That was before the integration, but even then I remembered being so intrigued by the books I read. Never did I encounter a character who looked like me. None of them looked like my father or my family, and they certainly didn't do the things that we did or talk the way that we did. You can't understand what it's like to not have characters like this if you've always had them at your disposal. The white girls I went to school with had friends like them to talk to, but if their friends didn't understand, they could pick up a book and find a girl who looked just like them. These characters allowed them see humans like them and gave them an avenue to figure things out for themselves. I never had even a fictional world to retreat to.

I reflected on the times when my brother and I would sit and imagine our adult lives and what they might be like. We would talk of the things we might accomplish. My father only made it as far as the first grade. He had to drop out of school and work or pick cotton. This enabled him to contribute financially as well care for his younger siblings. My mother made it to eleventh grade before she dropped out after having her first child. But they both saw the importance of education and wanted to see a better life for their children. They bought us these encyclopedias, called *The Story of Mankind,* and my brother and I would sit for hours reading chapters out of those books.

The first time that I did come across a book that I could relate to was in eighth grade. It was by the author, Annie Moody and called, *Coming of Age in Mississippi.* It was one of the few books about black people in our library. I was fascinated from page one. The places it spoke about were places that I had heard of. The things that the author talked about were things that I had heard my parents talk about. My parents were from Mississippi so there was quite a bit of overlap and similarities. And what was even more unbelievable was the author wrote about the events of the early 1960s. The realities that I lived through, she had the courage to not only speak about, but to write down. It blew me away.

I thought a lot about that book during that pivotal point when I was pregnant with my second child. I thought about how much I respected her assertive response to the heartache of that time. I knew that I needed to foster this sense of assertiveness within myself as well. Once I had my child, I felt the thirst to prove myself. I went back to school. I went to day school and night school, anything to catch up on the credits I needed for graduation. And as graduation neared, I didn't think, "I've made it," or "I'm done now;" I thought about college.

I remember one Sunday afternoon sitting in front of the television with my brother after one of his football teams had lost again. We were teenagers, my second child was a toddler, and we started talking about college. I shared with him that I wanted to go to college, but I also longed to go somewhere with a large black community, and even though there were plenty of black people in Mississippi, I wanted to go somewhere else, somewhere new and exciting like maybe Washington DC. I also was realizing that I had a longing to learn about illnesses and the causes. My grandfather, Malcolm Smiley died before I was born, but I knew he had cancer of an internal organ, and I always longed to know more. I had read somewhere that they called Washington DC "Chocolate City". There were so many black people. My brother suggested that I apply to Howard University. As we researched and did whatever we needed for information (these were the days before Google), we went to those encyclopedias. The Story of Mankind. Sure enough there was information on Howard University. I found their address and wrote to them requesting an application.

Upon receipt of the application, I excitedly filled it out and paid the $25 application fee. I waited, and waited. Finally, I got the return letter and tore it open on the spot. I was accepted. This was the start of new path. After a small stint at Howard University, I transferred to the University of the District of Columbia. By this time, I had two of my children living with me in Washington DC. The transfer to the UDC allowed me to become a nurse in three years, and I knew that this was the path I wanted to take. I had found my way, and it turned out that those encyclopedias helped me to do so. I think about those books all the time, and how they allowed me to travel even when I couldn't physically do so. In my physical existence I had been to Mississippi numerous times on family vacations. But those books allowed me to go so much farther.

Once I received my degree in Nursing, I started wondering again. I wanted to understand my abilities and what my mission in this life was. I had read *Philosophical Consciencism* by Kwame Nkrumah, and it theorized about the interactions between mind and body and surmised that the mind can manifest thoughts into concrete matter. In other words, thinking and visualization truly are the key to making things happen. That's how I've gotten as far as I've gotten, and I continue to move forward.

My purpose is to move forward in life, to be alive, to thrive and live life fully. I long to empower all of the people I meet so that they understand and work toward balancing of their mental, physical and spiritual selves. This is so that they can acknowledge and accept their worth. I want them to realize or remember that there is a place for them on this planet and in this universe, but it can so easily be forgotten or lost; but it's no accident that any of us is here.

We all have our challenges in life. Things get hard, times go dark, and it seems like paths are closed off to us. But life gives us what we can handle. It gives us what we need to emerge at the other end, a shining, brilliant diamond, or sapphire or ruby. Those stones couldn't exist without adverse conditions. They move through those stresses and show up as the most beautiful gems we could imagine. And in fact we couldn't imagine it, if we didn't see it with our own eyes. My goal for me and for anyone reading this is to accept change and allow room for it. Keep an open mind and heart by looking, seeing and embracing what comes rather than pushing it away.

"Where a woman rules, streams run uphill"
– Ethiopian Proverb

Biography

Professional Nurse Author and Entrepreneur that has spanned decades. Willa is a mother of three, a grandmother of five, a sibling to a clan of nine other with a host of other extended family. A goal in life is to engage in it, continue to evolve, with it and practice self-care as a habit.

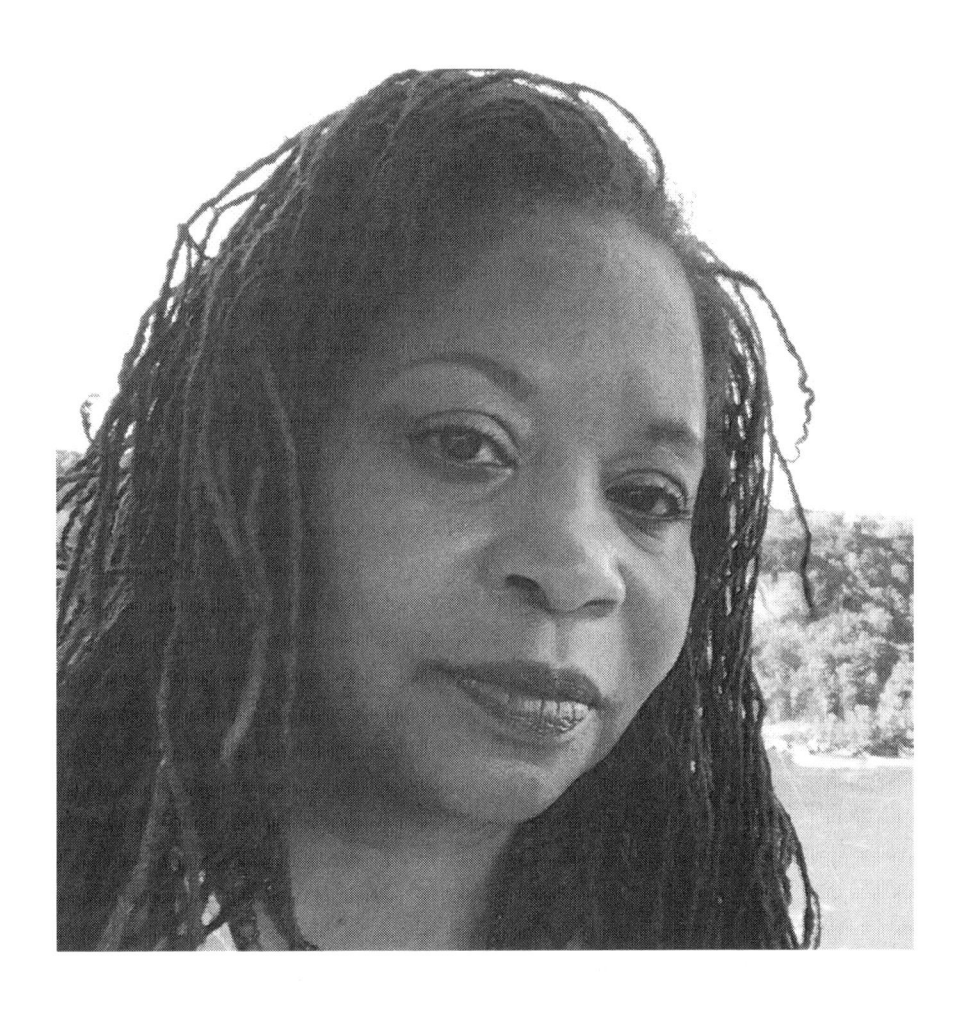

Against the Odds

By Kerine Dent-Alston, RN

If you sent two people into the same clothing store with the same budget on the same day, chances are these two people are going to emerge from that store in totally different outfits. There's even a chance that one will come out looking absolutely stunning and the other will look like she got dressed in the dark. If that's the case, you wouldn't look at the poorly dressed person and think, "Well, they just didn't have the same opportunity." You couldn't think that because everything about their circumstances was the same. It's not so much the tier of the store that you sent them into. You could send two people into a Goodwill, or you could send them into a Neiman Marcus, and the truth is if you have style, you'll come out looking good in either case. If you don't, you won't. It doesn't matter how expensive the components of your wardrobe. If you don't have that guiding fashion sense, money can't save you. But the real gem here is that if you do have that guiding sensibility, lack of money or resources can't hurt you, either.

This scenario is an everyday example of a very real concept. We all come into this world with a particular wardrobe already in place. Those are our circumstances. And we all come into this world with the ability to utilize our guiding sensibility (God) if we choose to ask for His assistance. Maybe we get to enter this world with a wardrobe that we really like. The quality of clothes is high, the materials are rich and the durability is unparalleled. But more often than not, we enter into a world where the wardrobe is lacking. Fabrics are worn thin, garments have holes and the colors are fading. In this situation, it's so easy to blame the wardrobe when we're dressed shabbily. It's so easy to get angry and stay angry because our choices are just so bad. I get it - where's the fairness in one person being born with a Nordstrom gift card and the other being born with a Savers gift card? It's not fair.

But what I've learned, and what I hope to share, is that this life is not fair and it's not meant to be. Not all of us get a fair shot just because we show up. The real beauty of life is in transformation and seeing how much we can do despite what we do or don't have at the outset. We are here to see what we can do with what we have. The real magic is turning a whole lot of nothing into something remarkable. Think about how we approach Halloween. No one wants to spend a lot of money on a Halloween costume that you wear for one night. So, what do we do? We go to Goodwill, looking for cheap odds and ends that we can turn into a cool costume. We dig around in the back of our closets and see if we can find some treasures in our friends' collections. Now, think about that feeling when you actually find some gems from that hodgepodge of secondhand clothes and forgotten items. Think about that feeling when you've spent hardly anything, yet you have a costume that is a showstopper.

That's what we are here to do. Most likely, life has given you a hodgepodge of detritus to deal with, unbecoming circumstances that were preordained long before you were even a glimmer in your parents' eyes. You can take what you end up with and get angry about it, or you can take it and see what you can turn it into. If you approach it all with an open mind and an eye for possibility, rather than a feeling of being slighted, you have an opportunity to make something magical. And it's in that transformation where our true purpose lies.

Now don't get me wrong. I'm not saying any of this is easy. The wardrobe that I was given to start out with was a far cry from any store you'd find in the mall. I grew up in the ghetto where I saw things no child should see. From the time that I was eight years old until I was twelve, I was molested by a person who was supposed to love and protect me but, instead, only traumatized me.

What that did to me went beyond the physical. It seeped into my spirit and made me feel worthless to the core. I thought that I had done something wrong, and I blamed myself for what was happening to me. But I didn't feel like I could talk about it, so I internalized all my feelings. I felt like it wouldn't be happening to me if I didn't deserve it, and the last thing I wanted to do was hurt my mom by bringing it up. So, instead I tried to be better, hoping the problem would correct itself, but of course that didn't stop any of it. I did write a letter addressed to my dad articulating what I felt to the best of my ability. I never gave it to him; I hid it away in my pants pocket. It was more for my own processing and not to actually give to him, but my mother did end up finding that letter years later. She confronted him and asked him if it was true, and he admitted to it. After being married for so many years, she left him. It meant a lot that she sided with me and not him, but the damage had already been done. I was filled to the brim with pain, so I shoved it down, as deep as it would go. I thought that meant it was gone, but I was wrong.

Suffice it to say, I had not been dealt a winning hand. And my initial reaction was exactly what you'd expect. I got angry. I got really angry. I was a naturally smart kid, so I started out in school doing really well. But once I started stuffing down all my anger toward being molested, my grades fell. I didn't care. I saw a world that was out to get me, one that was being hard on me for no apparent reason. So, I was defiant. I lived recklessly and did what I wanted because I allowed the devil to trick me into thinking that no one cared what happened to me. So, I didn't care either. I layered myself in an untouchable and indifferent attitude and became tough. It wasn't unlike how scar tissue develops over a wound and takes on a different consistency.

I had three kids by the time I was eighteen years old, by someone who did not value our children or me. I had dropped out of school, and I wasn't hanging out with the best crowd. One night, I went out with the cousin of my children's father and there was a crime committed that could have landed me some time in prison. I was charged as an accessory after the fact because I was there and didn't report it, which, in the state of South Carolina, is a felony. I was thrown in jail and stayed for thirty days. During that time, I couldn't see my children. I was alone and cold. All I could do was think.

That was my turning point. Sitting there in that cold cell, miles away from my children, I found God - or maybe God found me. It was like He had hit the pause button on my life and was sitting me down for a stern talking to. He was trying to get me to stop, stay still and take a deeper look at what I was doing and where I was headed. I knew in my heart that if I had been home where I should've been, I would have never ended up in that predicament. But I wasn't home because my relationship with my children's father was toxic and abusive, and I was in financial trouble. I tried to console myself by telling myself that my circumstances put me in that situation, and that it had nothing to do with me.

But God forced me to look at that again. Yes, the relationship was toxic and abusive. Yes, I was in financial trouble. Yes, things weren't going well at all, but I was the one who had chosen how I responded. And because I was so full of anger and indifference, I chose a step that separated me from my kids, ostracized me from the community and landed me somewhere that was not the kind of place where I wanted to be sitting as a mother who loved her kids so deeply. But the bright part of that realization was, as bad of a choice as I had made, that choice was mine. Which meant, if I had the power to make a bad choice, I also had the power to make a good choice. If I continued down this path of darkness, I'd have to choose it, and I was not going to purposefully choose that type of path.

My bail was set at $1500, and yes, my mom and dad could have bailed me out, but they opted to give me some tough love instead. While in jail, I met another young lady with circumstances similar to mine. As we talked and prayed together with five other young women, this lady promised me that when she was released, she would pay my bail. It was a sign from God when she stuck to her promise. So, when I got out after thirty days, the first thing I did was call my mom, apologize for my disobedience and ask her to come and get me from South Carolina as soon as I was finished with court. If I was going to change, I was going to have to change my environment. The unfortunate circumstances that I had been given were mine and mine alone to change. My anger was simply perpetuating the cycle. My goal now was to pick up the pieces, look around at what I had that was good - my children, my family, my mind, and my strength - and create something positive from that.

I went home about six months later, ready to move down a totally different path. I was given two years probation and wasn't actually allowed to leave the state. But for me, it was imperative that I change my environment and go home. Staying in South Carolina, even if it was part of the probation, was only going to keep me engulfed in negative influences and habits. So instead, I went back home to Rochester, pregnant with my third child and reported to the probation office there so that there'd be a record that I was not running or hiding but simply changing my life. I made sure that I had a job within two weeks of being home, and that I was headed down a healthy path. When a representative from South Carolina finally did come searching for me with a warrant for my arrest for breaking my probation in that state, I had my life in order, and everything ended up working out. For me, the way everything fell together at this point proved to be another sign that when you trust God, things work themselves out.

I finished a CNA program and was accepted into an LPN program that would take me ten months to complete. Shortly after completing the LPN program, I was accepted into a two-year RN program that I also completed. Today, I continue to provide patients with bedside care, which I thoroughly enjoy. I am also the proud co-owner of a travel nurse staffing agency called StatRN. I pray daily and seek God's advice whenever I feel weak. I trust Him completely to get me through anything that life can throw at me. I made sure that I changed my circle and continue to surround myself with only people whom I trust. It's so important to surround yourself with good people who share your values and who you can rely on to pick you up rather than steer you down a dark path. Just like anything else, the people you interact with and confide in are choices. You choose who gets to be in your circle, and it's a privilege to be one of those people. For so long, I had felt worthless because of what happened to me, so it didn't seem like there was value in being in my circle. But God showed me that this wasn't true at all.

Being abused as a child causes you to lose that feeling of empowerment. You start to think that the apathy and lack of care with which you were treated is the truth. So, you stop valuing yourself and think you do not deserve to be surrounded by people with integrity and standards. That's something that I had to learn to take back. It's not a luxury to hang out with good people; it's a priority.

I now have six kids, and I look at all of them and what God has given me, and I am so grateful. I'm close with all of them, and I make sure that they know I'm here for them no matter what. I remember, all too well, what it was like to be so angry and to feel so betrayed, and I do everything in my power to make sure the opposite is true for them. They have been my motivating factor all these years, and continue to inspire me daily.

I also have parents who love me and have been there for me no matter what. I am grateful for the tough love they've given me because I'm not sure if I would be who I am today without it. For so long, I was angry with them for what happened to me, but through being a parent, I can see now that their response was love. As an angry teen, I imagined that I'd feel better if they made my abuser feel the pain that I had felt. But as a parent, I now understand that there is no reward in creating pain in another person, even if that seems like the answer in the moment. The reward and healing comes through love, strength and empowerment. If they had focused on causing him pain instead of loving and strengthening me, they would've been consumed with those negative emotions. That wouldn't have made them better parents to me even though at the time I just desperately wanted them to take some action. I understand now that I had tied their reaction and inability to hurt my abuser back to what they felt for me. Because they didn't do what I wanted, I assumed they weren't as angry as I was. But the truth was that they were just as angry as me, possibly angrier. Just like I'd be furious if anything like this happened to my children. But what they knew and what I had yet to learn, was that the pain was not for them to deal out. That was God's job, and this situation had to be handled God's way. I am forever grateful for everything they've done and continue to do for my children and me.

My life isn't perfect now, and I'm not perfect either, by any stretch. But I know something now that I didn't understand back then. I know that no matter what happens to you, no matter what you start with, or what you're going through, you can always change it. There is always a choice somewhere, embedded in the mess of it all. You are not defined by your past. You do the best you can at a moment in time. But your "best" is not a stagnant truth. That night I went to jail, the best I could do was get in that car. But then I grew. I spoke to God. I found my way, and my "best" moved up a notch. I grew a little closer to my true potential. I realized that I define my future. I determine when my "best" becomes a little better.

That's also not to say that I've forgotten my roots. They will always be a part of my story, but they are just that – a part. They are not the entire story. Friends and family who knew me when I was young sometimes see me today and are so impressed with how far I've come. And that's actually what's so magical about a person who starts out with tough circumstances. It's just like seeing a seed that has taken root on some rocky mountainside with hardly any soil. When you see a tree like that - emerging from sheer rock on a mountainside battered by wind and weather - when you see a healthy, thriving tree growing from that, you can't help but feel a little bit of magic. And you know that God really must've wanted that tree in the world, because there's no way it should have survived, never mind thriving.

And so that's why my purpose is to share the message that circumstances are simply that – circumstances. You can just as easily call them tools or clothes in a wardrobe. We all get to take what we've been given and to turn it into something better. I've shared this message in my career as a nurse. I've seen those patients who are full of anger and are walled off from the world, and I sit with them and say, "We need to have a chat." I've cried with patients and their families because we've witnessed those "aha" moments together, those moments that caused the change. I know I've made a difference in people's lives because I don't judge. My past informs me that there's always room for change. The people who make the biggest difference take whatever they're given and make use of it for good. You've got to just love yourself enough to go through it because what's on the other end is always worth it.

The thriving tree on the mountainside is worth it. That stellar Halloween costume created from nothing is worth it. And just like me, you're worth it. We all are.

Anything or anyone who can emerge out of the ashes, against all odds, is absolutely worth it. And whatever we've learned along the way, and can share with others, is the purpose God intended.

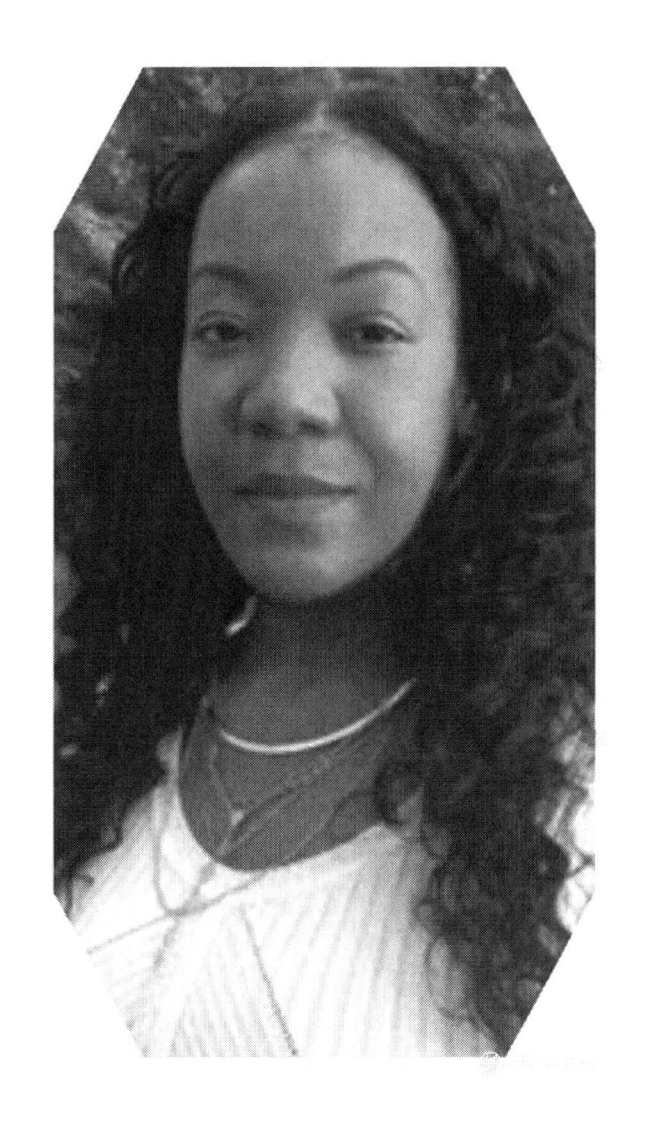

Made in the USA
San Bernardino, CA
03 January 2020